Conversations in Later Life

A Cognitive Analytic Approach to Aging Well

Edited by Michelle Hamill, Ellen Khan and Paul Catlin

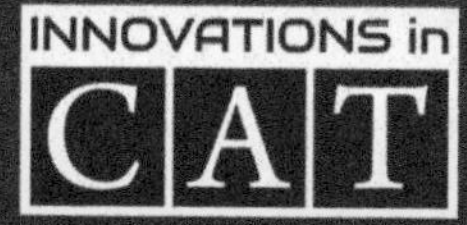

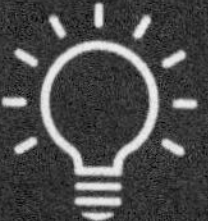

Conversations in Later Life:
A Cognitive Analytic Approach to Aging Well

Published by:

Pavilion Publishing and Media Ltd
Blue Sky Offices, 25 Cecil Pashley Way,
Shoreham by Sea, West Sussex, BN43 5FF

Tel: +44 (0) 1273 434 943
Email: info@pavpub.com
Web: www.pavpub.com

Published 2024

A catalogue record for this book is available from the British Library.

ISBN: 978-1-80388-399-1

Pavilion Publishing and Media is a leading publisher of books, training materials and digital content in mental health, social care and allied fields. Pavilion and its imprints offer must-have knowledge and innovative learning solutions underpinned by sound research and professional values.

Editors: Michelle Hamill, Ellen Khan and Paul Catlin
Cover design: Phil Morash, Pavilion Publishing and Media Ltd
Page layout and typesetting: Emma Dawe, Pavilion Publishing and Media Ltd
Printing: Independent Publishers Group (IPG)

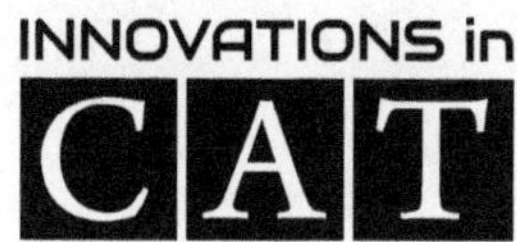

Available now in the *Innovations in CAT* series:

Creativity and Mental Health
(edited by Yvonne J. Stevens)

Innovative Practice in Forensic Settings
(edited by Jenny Marshall and Jamie Kirkland)

Working Relationally with Children and Young People
(edited by Nick Barnes and Lee Crothers)

Reflective Practice in Forensic Settings
(edited by Jenny Marshall and Jamie Kirkland)

'We belong and grow in a continuing web of relationships, with others and the outside world.'

Dr Anthony Ryle, in conversation
with Elizabeth Wilde McCormick, July 2011

To the many older adults and families
who have shared such wisdom, creativity
and resilience with us over the years.

Acknowledgements

Our deepest gratitude to family members, friends and colleagues who have sustained our commitment to this book, and we are very grateful to all of you for sharing your personal and professional insights. In particular, we would like to thank Dr Line Sagfors, Jane Sweetman, Dr Aisleen Keena, Dr Navi Nagra and Manjumitra Johannessen. Thank you for taking the time to read and re-read the drafts to form this book. All of you have left your mark.

Contents

Acknowledgements

Preface

About the editors

Contributors

Chapter 1: Setting the scene
Michelle Hamill and Ellen Khan 11

Chapter 2: The dance of relating in later life
Elizabeth Wilde McCormick 23

Chapter 3: Mapping a lifetime of stories
Steve Potter 47

Chapter 4: Finding a compassionate life story
Alistair Gaskell 69

Chapter 5: Who am I really? A CAT reflection on retirement
Henrietta Batchelor 89

Chapter 6: Once upon a time in Stepney – the legacy of complex trauma
Paul Catlin 121

Chapter 7: When health changes – caring and being cared for
Ellen Khan and Michelle Hamill 133

Chapter 8: Approaching the end – loss, mortality, and new beginnings in later life
Kitty Clark-McGhee and Emma Forde 155

Afterword

Appendix 1: The Psychotherapy File

Appendix 2: The Psychosocial Checklist

Appendix 3: Glossary of Key CAT terms

References

Preface

'Old age is a stage of our life, which, like all its other stages, has its own face, its own atmosphere and temperature, its own joys and sorrows. We have, like all our younger brothers, our own task, which gives meaning to our existence... in order to fulfil one's purpose in old age and cope with one's task, one must agree with old age and with everything that it brings with itself, one must say 'yes' to it... it would be wretched and sad to surrender solely to this process of decline and not see that old age has its good sides, its advantages, its comforts, and joys.'

Hymn to old age
Hermann Hesse (1952)

Across the world, people are living longer today than at any other time in history. How can we be enabled to live into our later years – crucially, in better health – and what does it mean to age well? The answers to these questions are multifaceted and research from around the world offers insights into how this can be achieved. A key factor to better health is improving mental health, at all ages. Our goal with this book is to offer a practical way of helping to understand and optimize emotional well-being in later life for anyone interested in this topic. We hope it will be of interest to people across their later years as well as clinicians working in later-life settings. Throughout the book, we will offer insights, exercises and tools drawing on research related to emotional developments in later life and Cognitive Analytic Therapy (CAT) that can offer a pragmatic approach to better emotional awareness and psychological health as we age. The exercises can be done alone or with a supportive friend, family member or person you trust. If you are a clinician working in later-life settings, the exercises may help you to focus on thinking relationally with the people you are working with.

For some people, the basic building blocks of healthier aging may seem obvious – a better diet, exercise, supportive relationships, and having a sense of purpose in life. However, many of us are remarkably good at not doing the things that can help us the most, getting stuck in unhelpful patterns and habits, and compromising the possibilities for better health and well-being. For some people, earlier or lifelong experiences of neglect, feeling inadequate, stuck or undeserving may mean that attending to these basics is hard, and often unmanageable. Compassion for oneself and others can feel very difficult, and expectations for a meaningful life may be low. For others, the adjustments that can arise in later life may mean that once-reliable coping strategies no longer work, triggering feelings of despair and worry. Later life can be a time when coping strategies are challenged by losses and transitions, which resonate with earlier experiences of distress and vulnerability, destabilizing emotional well-being. For many, the thought of getting older brings up worry and fears about illness, decline and dependency, which can get in the way of living life well, in the present. However, aging is by no means a simple downward trajectory of doom and gloom. The latter stages of life also bring unique opportunities and perspectives. It is possible to live a fulfilling and meaningful life in the advancing years, and discovering ways to confront and overcome fears of aging is central to this.

This book has its roots in three seminal books. First, is Liz Mc Cormick's *Change for the Better* (McCormick, 2017), a self-help book in its fifth edition, which guides readers through managing emotional distress and improving relationships, drawing on CAT and mindfulness. Second, is Laura Sutton and Jason Hepple's *Cognitive Analytic Therapy and Later Life* (Hepple & Sutton, 2004), which applied CAT understandings to later life for the first time in 2004, challenging the double pessimism that is all-too-frequently associated with both later life and mental distress. Finally, there is Steve Potter's *Therapy with a Map* from 2020. Drawing on these books, with Liz and Steve's personal reflections and insights, multiple perspectives of CAT, along with research into healthier aging and theories of emotional regulation in later life, we will offer ideas to help you review and subsequently revise relationship patterns and habits that may be no longer useful, within the changing context of aging. To succeed at this, part of this journey will involve learning what gets in the way of you doing what matters to you. Long-held patterns, which may go unquestioned or which are assumed to be fixed, can get in the way of our efforts to change and discover new possibilities for living a more fulfilled life. By developing a deeper understanding of yourself, within your life context and relationships, you can better recognize when you are getting stuck and start to do things differently, regardless of age.

As an integrative and time-limited psychological therapy, CAT brings together ideas and understanding from different therapies into one user-friendly and effective, evidence-based treatment (ACAT, undated) for a wide variety of mental health problems. It offers a lifespan model of growth and development that views every person as a 'work in progress' and that, regardless of age, personal growth and change for the better are possible. It focuses on personal concerns and is suitable for anyone interested in exploring their relational patterns within the context of their lives and experiences. It is not primarily concerned with traditional psychiatric symptoms, syndromes or diagnostic labels, and it can be applied to a wide range of emotional difficulties. It aims to help people find their own language for their experiences and set manageable goals to bring about change (Ryle & Kerr, 2020).

Throughout this book, we will draw on CAT tools, along with theories of emotional development and regulation in later life, to show how better health can be supported. We aim to offer a safe structure to support self-reflection, which can help with changing old habits and patterns that are no longer helpful and may be contributing to distress. A relational understanding shows us that what we do and the choices we make have their roots in past relationships and experiences, and that our actions will result in reactions in others. Our early life experiences shape us and the people that we become, setting up expectations with longstanding effects that persist through life. At some point, we will all face disappointments, failure or rejection. Relationships will end, we get sick and eventually we all die – no matter how much some of us try to deny these realities. Trying to pretend life is any other way only results in a rude awakening and makes life's inevitable pain worse when it comes. So, while we can't avoid the pain that is an inescapable part of life – as much as we may want to – we can learn to understand and manage painful experiences in ways that better serve our health and well-being.

CAT offers a framework to better understand who we are, with the courage to anticipate challenges, attend to fears, and remain open to learning, including in the face of pain. It offers a way to pause, step back and observe what is arising, and to make choices about how we respond in ways that don't make situations worse. We will provide in this book ideas for developing a more compassionate self-awareness and an improved ability to make choices about how we react to challenging situations, along with suggestions for how to manage difficult feelings and set realistic goals for change. While developing self-awareness through guided self-help differs from being in therapy, if you are interested in understanding emotional and relational issues in later life, this book can offer a way to do this at your own pace. The book may also be of interest if you are working in later-life settings or are supporting a person in their later years, and you wish to gain a better understanding of what may be contributing to their distress. We hope that it can offer ideas, including adapting the exercises to do together where language, education, health-related or other barriers to self-help may arise.

As accredited clinical psychologists and CAT psychotherapists, working across a range of settings – including older adult mental health services and private practice in the UK, along with personal experiences of aging and later life – we aim to provide evidence-based information and advice about aging well and coping when challenges arise in later years. Our work is informed by international experts in their respective fields of older adult mental health and emotional well-being, alongside the real experts – the older people and their families who inspire and teach us. It goes without saying that great diversity exists between individuals in later life, and there is no 'one-size-fits-all' approach to managing distress. While everyone's experience is unique, we believe this approach offers the flexibility to meet different individual needs. CAT is a hopeful model, and we want to convey this hope through the stories in this book. This is certainly what we have experienced in our clinical practice, and in our lives, over many years. It is never too late to engage in the work of aging and never too late to change. Attending to later life within the context of your whole life's journey to this point, with all its joys and sorrows, can help you to derive meaning and purpose as you continue to age, right until the end of life. Seeing the changes that are possible, regardless of age, and the resilience of people in their later years across our work settings, is a privilege.

How this book works

In this book, we bring together different voices within the field of CAT. Together, and using CAT ideas, the different writers offer both personal and professional reflections on a relational approach to understanding health and later-life challenges. CAT is a dynamic, creative and playful approach. What follows is a range of perspectives from the different chapter's authors, of how the theory can be used to help people in real life, offering the flexibility to tailor interventions according to different preferences and needs. While each writer has their own unique perspectives and style, we all are bound together in our use and appreciation of how CAT can support better health. This book will offer opportunities for readers, including clinicians and others interested in supporting a person in their later years, to develop relational awareness through guided self-reflection and through clinical case material to come to new insights about later life and its possibilities. Although the book is best read chronologically to get an understanding of CAT ideas and concepts and how they can be applied, different chapters may also offer insights on their own, given each author's unique voice and perspective. Chapters two and three aim to give the reader the 'nuts and bolts' of CAT and its core concepts. These are followed by chapters which illustrate these ideas further in practice, related to particular transitions and challenges that can arise in later life. If a chapter does not resonate or feel relevant, feel free to skip to the next one. Some chapters may require re-reading if the ideas and concepts are new, while others may connect and make sense straightaway. In each chapter, you will see exercises to help you to reflect, along with tools and ideas to support change. Have a pen and paper nearby to try these as you read. This will help with self-reflection and developing skills of relational awareness, alone or with someone else.

With respect to the limits of self-help, Liz helpfully summarizes some important key points in her book *Change for the Better*, which we repeat with her permission here. It is important to note that some problems and difficulties may require professional help, from a therapist or medical professional. While common symptoms including disturbed sleep, headaches, fatigue, pain and digestive issues may be the result of emotional and psychological distress, they can also be caused by medical conditions that require their own treatments. Please do not dismiss or ignore these experiences. If depression or anxiety are significant, or if any problems are more severe or prolonged, please seek appropriate professional advice, guidance and support. While some factors can be managed at an individual level, offering many opportunities for better health, other factors require systemic, economic and culture-wide policy changes so that everyone can benefit. Many problems in life are driven by social and political factors, far beyond the control of any one individual to overcome – poverty, poor housing, unemployment, discrimination, the impact of climate change, living in exile or being displaced due to conflict. These experiences drive poor health outcomes and result in significant distress . While CAT offers a means by which to make sense of such social and political factors within the context of a person's life, the appropriate actions will require political and collective change, far beyond the scope of this book.

Chapter 1 introduces some key theories and research related to emotional regulation and development in later life.

Chapter 2 outlines CAT in more detail, giving the reader an insight into developing an understanding of oneself and where change may be possible, along with ideas for looking after yourself and managing emotional distress.

Chapter 3 explains the CAT tools of mapping, showing how this process can offer a way to visually draw out relational patterns that are no longer working, which can be a powerful means to develop self-awareness and areas to change.

Chapter 4 explores the way that critical and judgemental narratives about ourselves are formed through life experiences and cultural forces and how we can come to a more compassionate understanding.

Chapter 5 offers some reflections on retirement and how the loss of formal work may impact individuals and challenge their identity when they relinquish their 'work self'.

Chapter 6 shares a personal account of developing new understandings of earlier life traumas through CAT in later life.

Chapter 7 explores the changing nature of relationships when care is required as a result of changing health, both from the perspective of finding oneself in a caring role or needing care from another person.

Chapter 8 invites a conversation about life endings and how we relate to them, particularly exploring how we experience death, dying and mourning alongside an increased closeness to our mortality as we age.

The chapters that lie ahead aim to be thought provoking and helpful. At times, the process of developing self-awareness may feel challenging. We hope that you can take your time, stop, and, most of all, not give up. Change is possible and it is never too late. We can become better observers of ourselves and each other as we age, and we can learn more compassionate and accepting ways of reacting and responding, to live well, right up until the end of our lives.

About the editors

Michelle Hamill is a consultant clinical psychologist and CAT practitioner and supervisor who has worked in the NHS for more than twenty years in the field of older adult mental health, memory clinics and dementia care. She has a particular interest in relationship-based psychological therapies and has co-authored a self-help book for carers of people with dementia: *How to Help Someone with Dementia.*

Ellen Khan is a principal clinical psychologist who has worked in the NHS for sixteen years. Ellen trained as a clinical psychologist at University College London and, since qualifying in 2013, has always worked with older people, people with dementia and their carers. As a clinical psychologist, Ellen draws on a number of therapeutic approaches, but particularly values CAT and the richness it offers. Ellen is a CAT practitioner and CAT supervisor and especially enjoys using CAT to work with early-life trauma and with carers of people with dementia.

Paul Catlin is a writer, activist and part-time lecturer of Anglo-Nigerian heritage. He is a longtime resident of the East End of London. Paul is currently engaged in fulfilling a lifetime ambition to write memoir – *Child of an Uncertain Future* – a sequel to the acclaimed novel *City of Spades*, in which the author Colin MacInnes chronicles his friendship with Paul's migrant father and the prevailing racial climate in post-war Britain.

About the editors

Contributors

Elizabeth Wilde McCormick is a founder and life member of ACAT, where, from the early 1980s, she was a psychotherapist, supervisor, trainer and, for many years, a trustee. Her background is in transpersonal and humanistic psychology, social psychiatry, sensorimotor psychotherapy and Cognitive Analytic Therapy. She is the author of several self-help psychological books including: *Surviving Breakdown; Living on the Edge; Your Heart and You* (with Dr Leisa Freeman) and *Change for the Better*, a CAT self-help book which is now in its fifth edition. The third book in her fictional 'Dr Max' trilogy was published in autumn 2023.

Steve Potter is a past chairperson and life member of ACAT. He values CAT as an integrative and relational framework for psychotherapy with individuals, groups and in reflective practice. He helped establish the International Cognitive Analytic Therapy Association and was its first chair. His early career was in therapy groups, social group work and teaching social psychology to youth and community workers. He was Director of Counselling at the University of Manchester and helped establish a CAT-based service. He has taught many courses, facilitates individual supervision and practices psychotherapy privately. He has written two books on psychotherapy and several articles and chapters.

Alistair Gaskell trained in clinical psychology at the University of East London in the early 1990s and in CAT at St Thomas's Hospital in the early 2000s. He has been practicing as an NHS psychologist for more than thirty years. He has a longstanding interest in the social and cultural context of psychotherapy and mental health, and is currently studying for a medical humanities MA at Birkbeck College. He writes from personal as well as professional experience of mental health problems.

Henrietta Batchelor is a Life Member of ACAT and is currently Chair of the ACAT Ethics Committee. She has a background in educational psychology research, teaching and relationship psychotherapy before she trained as a CAT psychotherapist and supervisor working in adult mental health in various settings. She retired in 2012 from her post as Consultant Psychotherapist in the Women's Health Psychology Service in Northumbria Healthcare NHS Trust, and has since worked in independent practice. She has published on supervision and post-natal depression, and has more recently written a chapter on CAT and ethics (*CAT and Ethics: Dare to be aware*) for the *Oxford Handbook of Cognitive Analytic Therapy* (2024).

Kitty Clark-McGhee is a principal clinical psychologist and CAT supervisor-in-training. She has worked as a clinician in the NHS for fourteen years, mostly in older adult mental health and dementia care. As a therapist, Kitty has trained in a range of therapeutic approaches, though her practice is most anchored by CAT, and the richness and accessibility in affords. Her research interests are methodologies of text analysis- discourse and narrative analysis- as a means to explore critical and alternative understandings of the construction and experience of selfhood.

Emma Forde is a senior clinical psychologist who has been using CAT to inform her work in the NHS for twelve years. She has an interest in trauma and adjustment, working with older people, people living with dementia, and their family members. Emma takes an integrative approach to therapeutic work and greatly values the opportunity and flexibility that CAT affords in making sense of our individual stories and difficulties in the therapy room and beyond.

Chapter 1: Setting the scene

Michelle Hamill and Ellen Khan

> *'Longer lives can, and I believe, will improve quality of life, at all ages... Now, there are problems associated with aging- diseases, poverty, loss of social status ... but the more we learn about aging, the clearer it becomes that a sweeping downward course is grossly inaccurate. Aging brings some rather remarkable improvements, increased knowledge, expertise, and emotional aspects of life improve.'*
>
> Laura Cartensen, Professor of Psychology and Founding Director, Stanford Center on Longevity, Stanford University, TED Talk[1]

People are living longer and societies around the globe are experiencing a historically unprecedented growth in the population of older adults (WHO, 2022). By the middle of this century, living to the age of one hundred will be more commonplace (Cartensen, 2022), and if current trends continue, by 2050 the global population over sixty-five years of age will double. These changes in life expectancy have been a remarkable achievement resulting from improvements in public health, food production, medicine and public education. However, they have happened so rapidly that social institutions, economic policies and social attitudes and norms, which evolved when people lived much shorter lives, are no longer sufficient or useful. Not only are they no longer useful, but these outdated policies and assumptions about aging can contribute to ageism and poor outcomes for health, well-being and relationships in later life.

In reviewing the literature, until quite recently, expectations about mental health in later life have been overwhelmingly negative (Cartensen, 2021) and it was assumed by and large that psychopathology and emotional disturbance increased with age in most older people (Pfeiffer, 1977). However, as time has gone on, research is steadily proving that these assumptions are incorrect and showing the numerous emotional

1 www.ted.com/talks/laura_carstensen_older_people_are_happier

advantages and developments in later life, some of which we will outline in this chapter and set the scene for the rest of the book.

What comes to mind when you think about aging and later life? For many people, the thought of aging is frightening, and some of us do our best to avoid thinking about it at all. Aging is not a disease. It is a multi-factorial process of natural change and people do not become old or elderly at any specific age. While aging cannot be avoided, many things can be done to maintain general good health and take some control over what happens as we age. Everyone ages differently, and there is huge variability in people in their later years, depending on life circumstances – those with financial security, a good education and a realistic attitude to aging tend to do best. It is not aging per se that negatively affects emotional well-being in later life. Rather, it is how aging is viewed, understood and managed that determines in large part how people feel as they get older.

Negative images of older age surround many of us, making it easy to believe that later life is simply a downward trajectory of doom and gloom. Generalized assumptions that older people are needy, incompetent and burdensome do not resonate with many older people, while ignoring age-associated vulnerabilities is equally problematic and can result in care and appropriate support being denied. While getting older can certainly bring challenges, decades of scientific and economic research across many countries and cultures shows not only that it is not all doom and gloom, but, on the contrary, that there are multiple emotional and social benefits associated with getting older (Cartensen, 2021), as outlined in this chapter. While we can't always change how others see aging in themselves or others, we can change how we respond and work with those common assumptions. Furthermore, where social policies have supported people to age 'well', positive economic and cultural contributions are possible, too, further challenging outdated and over-simplistic assumptions that so many hold about aging.

What does it mean to age successfully? While no single definition will satisfy everyone, the following seems apt: successful aging 'refers to reaching one's potential and arriving at a level of physical, social, and psychological well-being in old age that is pleasing to both self and others' (Gibson, 1995). Developmental psychologists Paul and Margret Baltes propose that aging well is possible through the successful enactment of certain strategies (Baltes & Baltes, 1993; Baltes, 1997), which help people make the most of their talents and opportunities, and to navigate around obstacles, depending on the specific personal, cultural, and societal circumstances they experience throughout their lives. The model focuses on gains and losses, alongside the great heterogeneity in aging and successful aging, and views successful mastery of goals in the face of losses endemic to advanced age as the result of the interplay of the three processes:

- *Selection* refers to the process individuals use to bring focus and prioritize goals as they age.
- *Optimization* is about maximizing the resources individuals currently possess (e.g., focusing more on crystalized versus fluid intelligence as we age).
- *Compensation* is about bringing in additional resources (e.g., using hearing or mobility aids to compensate for physical changes).

(Baltes & Cartensen, 1996)

Despite age-related changes, including illness and disabilities, older adults who are aging well can be enthused by life, engaged in meaningful relationships, have concern for the welfare of others, maintain optimism, and trust that they can continue to contribute and offer a legacy for others that is grounded in affirmation, irrespective of age. When challenges arise, they don't have to be transformed into mental roadblocks. Various studies (Valliant, 2002) have concluded that individual lifestyle, resilience and attitude may even contribute more to successful aging than genes, in many cases. The Nun's Study (Snowdon, 2008) showed that certain behaviours and traits in individuals may help to avert the clinical expression of some diseases, including Alzheimer's disease. Human beings are not fixed, although patterns of thinking and behaving can certainly feel rigid and dominating. These studies encourage us. It is possible to change unhelpful lifestyles, attitudes and relational patterns, and we will show how this is possible throughout the book.

The Blue Zones

The 'Blue Zone regions' are home to some of the oldest and healthiest people in the world and offer important insights into healthier aging. The term was first used by the author Dan Buettner (2012), who was studying areas of the world in which people live longer lives, notably in good health. They include Icaria, Greece; Ogliastra, Sardinia; Nagano and Okinawa,

Japan; Nicoya Peninsula, Costa Rica; and The Seventh-day Adventists in Loma Linda, California. Not only do people in these places reportedly live longer, but they also report lower chronic diseases, including dementia, cancer, cardiovascular disease, and stroke, and better mental health. While it is thought that genetics account for 20-30% of longevity, environmental influences, including diet and lifestyle, play a huge role in determining lifespan (Takata *et al*, 1987; Passarino *et al*, 2016; Hjelmborg *et al*, 2006). Although their lifestyles differ slightly, people from these places mostly eat a plant-based diet, exercise regularly, and get enough sleep. They also share strong family, social and faith-based networks along with having a life purpose or motivation to live including work, hobbies and relationships, all of which help to manage stress and recharge energy. Great emphasis is placed on community and social participation, and older adults are not made to feel like a burden to society. Instead, their unique and varied contributions to family over the generations and their communities are valued. Given the strong links between isolation and developing chronic disease conditions – from dementia to heart disease and poor mental health – the need for social connections is imperative when it comes to improving health across the lifespan.

You may want to note some thoughts down for this first exercise so that you can come back to them over time. This can help with starting to see where ideas, beliefs and motivations come from and their place in your life.

Exercise

- What motivates you daily?
- Where do these motivations come from?
- What brings you joy, satisfaction and pleasure?
- What interests you?
- What is important to you in life? What do you want more of in life?
- What are your main roles and relationships in life (employee, partner, parent, carer) and how do these motivate you?
- If you cannot do certain things in life anymore, perhaps due to age-related changes or other changes, are there other activities, relationships or interests, which are meaningful and that you could engage in?

As a relational model, CAT holds social connections at its heart. With its emphasis on social and cultural contexts when making sense of our identities, CAT can also facilitate more adaptive ways of being in the world, including attending to the impacts of harmful stereotypes and assumptions. Our lives and well-being are shaped by influences and factors beyond us and our relationships. Social, cultural and political factors are hugely influential. Our mental health is conditional on feeling valued and having a role in society and our communities, and negative assumptions about later life can have a powerful effect on people's self-esteem and mental health. If society is telling you that you are a burden and don't have any value, it can be hard to feel good about yourself and believe that you matter.

In contrast to the Blue Zones, age discrimination is present in many societies (WHO, 2021) leading to poorer health, social isolation, earlier deaths and costing economies billions. A report by the UN across fifty-seven countries found that half of all people held moderately or highly ageist attitudes (i.e., stereotypes and prejudice). In the UK, ageism is the most prevalent form of discrimination (Officer *et al*, 2020). Add discrimination due to race, sexual orientation, gender and disabilities into the mix and many older people face a perfect storm of their needs being discriminated against and denied. As a result, many societies are failing to benefit fully from the valuable resources that people in their later years can offer. Throughout the book, we will show how these social and cultural expectations play a significant role in our health and well-being. Being able to stand back, question and challenge incorrect and outdated assumptions and generalizations about aging will benefit everyone's health.

To date, the true costs and benefits of later life have been distorted by largely static views of what it means to age. Using rigorous scientific and economic research, the Stanford Centre on Longevity (Cartensen, 2022) calls for a shift from a purely deficit mindset, which solely laments the losses associated with aging, to the real economic and social contributions of older adults. In doing so, we can get a true account of the net costs and benefits of our current population structure and the many ways that adults in their later years add value and contribute to society. The AARP Longevity Economy Outlook (2016) evidence that adults aged fifty and older are a dominant force in the US economy. They project that the economic contributions of this cohort are set to triple by 2050, considering assets, wages, salaries, jobs created, consumer spending, taxes paid, and the market value of time spent caring and volunteering. Research also shows that many people experience good health and independence into their seventies and eighties, and cognitive trajectories vary widely, highlighting that the potential for longer working lives has more to do with ability, need, and interest, rather than age alone. New healthcare technologies and treatments also offer the hope of supporting independence and well-being in the advancing years. While everyone's life is unique, it is important to acknowledge a more balanced view of aging, as it is within this balanced perspective that aging and later life can be viewed realistically and fairly.

Psychological perspectives on aging

Although we have come a long way since then, Erik Erikson (1959; 1984; Erikson *et al*, 1986) was one of the first psychologists to develop a lifespan theory of psychosocial development, outlining the emotional tasks required at each major life stage, including later life. He proposed that, during each stage, we experience a 'psychosocial crisis' where the psychological needs of the individual conflict with the needs of society, and this could have a positive or negative outcome for that person's emotional well-being. Erikson's final stage begins at around age sixty-five and ends at death. He proposed that during this time we contemplate our accomplishments and can develop integrity if we see ourselves as leading a successful life, and central to this is acceptance. As Erikson reflected 'the acceptance of one's one and only life cycle as something that had to be' (Erikson, 1950, p268) and as 'a sense of coherence and wholeness' (Erikson, 1982, p65).

Erikson proposed that individuals who reflect on their lives and regret not achieving their goals will experience feelings of bitterness and despair. This is something we have experienced in our clinical settings. The process of life review, contemplation and acceptance is central to CAT's approach and ideas for how to do this will follow in the chapters ahead. While is it unrealistic to expect that we will achieve every goal and wish in life, it is possible and helpful to both attend to what was and what was not, with acceptance, thereby letting go of regret. As Liz writes in *Change for the Better* (McCormick, 2017, p11): 'We can breathe life into our experiences by observing thoughtfully the hand we have been dealt, accepting that we have done the best we could with what we had at the time, without judging or getting depressed. Acceptance is a start, and it is never too late to begin.'

Despite the limitations of his theory, to his credit, Erikson emphasized reciprocity across the life course, where older and younger people need each other to flourish, stating that 'Life doesn't make any sense without interdependence. We need each other, and the sooner we learn that, it is better for us all.' Intergenerational divides between younger and older adults feel increasingly polarized – politically, economically and culturally. Britain is one of the most age-segregated countries in the world (United For All Ages, 2017). The UK think tank 'United for All Ages' observes that the gulf between the ages is harmful on many levels, causing loneliness and exclusion, lack of trust, ageism and division. Loneliness is now one of the biggest threats to the physical and mental health of all generations. However, it doesn't have to be like this. More and more projects are enabling older and younger people to mix and share activities and experiences with multiple benefits, such as increased mutual understanding and tackling big issues like ageism, care, health and housing . Further social and political support is needed to continue this work to benefit everyone.

With regards to mental health and well-being in later life, while it may seem counterintuitive, study after study across many cultures shows that older people are often *more* satisfied with their lives than people in their middle and younger years (Regier *et al*, 1984; Shallcross *et al*, 2012). Except for the dementias, older adults have been found to display less psychological distress than at other ages (George *et al*, 1988; Blazer & Hybels, 2014). Contrary to popular opinion, when it comes to well-being, our lives do not represent an inevitable decline from our younger to our later years. Instead, the opposite is often true. Social scientists call this the 'paradox of aging': that improved psychological well-being is common despite the challenges and very real age-related losses that go with aging. Many studies (Mroczek & Kolarz, 1998) have found that, compared to younger adults, older adults report more positive emotional experiences and better subjective control over their emotions (Gross *et al*, 1997), along with more empathy (Sze *et al*, 2012) and gratitude (Chopik *et al*, 2019) and increased capacity for forgiveness (Cheng & Yim, 2008). Not only do these studies challenge assumptions about aging, they also challenge assumptions about well-being itself. Despite the declines in later life of the typically presumed factors associated with feeling good – health, social status, broad social networks, and high levels of social engagement – psychological well-being often improves.

Laura Cartensen *et al* have developed a theory based on many years of research with older adults across many countries and cultures to explain this 'paradox of aging' (Cartensen, 1992; 1993; 2006; Cartensen & Fredrickson,

1998; Cartensen *et al*, 2011). Their theory posits that recognizing that we won't live forever can, in one's later years, sharpen our focus on the here and now and on what really matters (Fung & Cartensen, 2004; Fung *et al*, 2001). It is also not the case, then, that increasing awareness of mortality causes unhappiness. As people age, goals change: there is more of an impetus to live in the moment, know what's important, invest in sure things, deepen relationships, and savour life. When we realize we don't have all the time in the world, our priorities shift. This can also be seen in people with terminal illnesses, of all ages. As a result, we take less notice of trivial matters, and invest more in emotionally important parts of life, and life gets better as a result. Goals shift from being more future-focused in middle life to goals realized in the present.

It is also not as simple to say that older people just tend to be happier. Rather a range of research studies show that older people tend to be less *unhappy* than younger people. Across race, gender and socioeconomic status, negative emotions were reported less frequently as people grew older, and, over time, individuals became less emotionally labile and more stable. Furthermore, emotional experiences appear to grow more complex with age. Older people report experiencing more mixed emotions including poignancy (Hershfield *et al*, 2008; 2013) – times that are joyful *yet also* bring a tear to one's eye – which in turn may increase gratitude. While anger, stress, frustration and anxiety appear to decrease with aging, sadness does not. Nor does sadness increase either. It has been suggested that sadness may be more valuable in later life than anger or anxiety, as it aids in sympathy and communication – valuable skills for many of the events faced in later life. Emotions, such as excitement, pride, calm and elation, have been found to generally remain stable across the lifespan. Only people in their advanced old age reported a slight decline in positive emotions (Charles *et al*, 2013).

Another developmental improvement associated with later life is increased acceptance. *Acceptance* – the ability to accept the reality of one's situation as it is – has been found to increase with age (Shallcross, *et al*, 2013). Learning the skills of acceptance forms the basis for many psychological approaches to better mental health. This is good news as, given that acceptance increases with age, this skill can be usefully drawn on to enhance well-being and manage difficult situations and feelings, which we will demonstrate throughout the book, and some of the exercises in the book can support you with this. Research has shown that greater acceptance in later life correlates with higher quality of life, despite objective challenges being faced (Butler & Ciarrochi, 2007). Acceptance involves a willingness to experience feelings without trying to change or avoid them. The idea of engaging more with negative emotions might seem counterintuitive, however the aim of acceptance is not to reduce difficult feelings, but rather to remain open to them without judgement. Emotions serve a purpose – they signal to us what we need, and they promote emotional intelligence and wisdom – so they should not be avoided or disregarded. However, all too often in life we have been taught to cope with painful feelings through avoidance. Research shows that approaching negative emotions with acceptance and without judgement helps them to diffuse (Campbell-Sills *et al*, 2006). Taking the example of sadness, as mentioned above, acceptance may play a meliorating role, preventing sadness from becoming overwhelming in the face of repeated losses in later life.

Despite the evidence that well-being and satisfaction improve as we age, many people still tend to dread growing older, holding firm to the belief that life satisfaction declines as we get older. Laura Cartensen suggests that, perhaps for many, we need to grow old ourselves before we celebrate the discoveries and benefits of this life stage that prove us wrong.

Exercise

- Think back to the beginning of the chapter. What images or words came to mind when you thought about aging?
- Have these changed over time, as you or other people you know have aged?
- Can you recall what you thought about aging and later life when you were younger?

If you ask many people ‘What does old age look like?’, they will probably think of ill-health, frailty, nursing homes and the loss of loved ones. This is a key part of the issue – our reasoning about aging can be faulty (Bell, 2019). When we evaluate our lives, we tend only to pay attention to a few aspects, and when it comes to thinking about later life, we tend to focus more on the negatives, which leads us to expect that life will be miserable. Research also shows that, by and large, people are poor predictors of their future well-being (Ubel *et al*, 2005). Specifically, people overestimate the impact and duration of negative emotions in response to loss. People without a given disability rate their expected quality of life significantly lower than people who are living with that disability. Researchers have demonstrated this gap for health conditions ranging from visual impairment and heart disease to asthma, dialysis, or living with a colostomy (Ubel *et al*, 2001; Baron *et al*, 2003). We seem to be poor at envisaging our capacity to adapt to declines in health. We also seem to forget that there may be other negatives associated with our middle years that we won't have to deal with anymore either – the rat race, doing a job we don't like or the pressures of working while child rearing and maybe caring for others too. Studies also show that older adults may be better at avoiding situations and people that make them feel bad (Mather, 2012; 2020; Mather & Cartensen, 2005). Who we spend time with has a major effect on our mood. Older adults tend to have more control over how they spend their time and whom they spend it with. Research has also found that social connections do not simply narrow due to bereavements and losses in later life, as assumed, rather these are proactively shaped and selectively pruned to support changing goals and become more emotionally meaningful over time (English & Cartensen, 2014).

However, reported developmental benefits aside, there is no getting away from the fact that life can be painful and getting older can throw up challenges and knock us off balance. It is with some of these challenges in mind that we write this book. We have found that CAT is well placed to collaborate therapeutically with older people and others in their lives, across a wide spectrum of issues that can present in later life. It offers a sensitive, flexible and versatile framework in which to explore people's rich life stories and the legacy of life events and relationships to bring about change, where required. It offers a coherent way of linking past and present, emphasizing the interpersonal and social context to find shared meaning and understanding across generational and cultural boundaries to manage distress in later life. CAT also attends carefully and explicitly to endings, sensitively addressing issues of intimacy and loss, which can underlie emotional distress, enabling conversations about how these experiences can be better managed. The chapters that follow will explore these ideas in greater detail.

Exercise

Before you read on, and to set the groundwork for making changes, the first step in this exercise is to start to develop non-judgemental self-awareness – the ability to observe your thoughts, feelings, sensations and reactions with increasing acceptance in the moment. Through increased self-awareness and recognition of where you are getting stuck, it becomes possible to try something new. Accepting every attempt and honouring your commitment to change, even when setbacks arise, is essential.

Start by getting comfortable in a quiet place where you won't be disturbed. Take a couple of minutes to focus on your breathing, close your eyes, become aware of any tension in your body, and let that tension go with each out-breath. Imagine a place where you can feel calm, peaceful and safe. It may be a place you've been to before, somewhere you've dreamed about going to, somewhere you've seen a picture of, or just a peaceful place you can imagine and create in your mind's eye. Notice the colours, the atmosphere, shapes, sounds and any sensations that you can bring to mind. Notice how this feels in your body and place your hand where you most connect with feelings of security and calm. You can return to this place anytime you want and, with practice, connecting here should come increasingly easily. It can help to choose a name for your safe place.

Anytime you notice you are becoming overwhelmed, ruminative, or disorganized in your thinking you can return to this calm, safe place. Once you are calm, try to note what the cause seemed to be. The better you become aware of situations or experiences that provoke or stir up difficult feelings and reactions, the more prepared you will feel to manage them.

Spending a few minutes each day, sitting quietly will also help with the development of self-awareness. Just try to notice whatever comes up for you – how you feel physically and emotionally, your stream of consciousness – and write everything down. Many of us give little time, if any, to reflecting on how we are feeling, and as such, when difficulties arise, we can quickly become overwhelmed or shut down. Becoming more aware of the changing nature of our experiences helps us to understand and manage these differently, where needed.

Summary

Later life brings many opportunities for emotional growth and developmental strengths, including increased acceptance and focus on life in the here and now. It is this enhanced tolerance and ability to accept feelings that offers hope and underpins how change and managing difficult feelings are not only possible in later life but are developmentally supported. These developments in emotional regulation can help when it comes to changing long-held and unhelpful patterns of avoiding and running away from feelings, and learning to care for what has been absent or neglected, thereby improving our emotional well-being. If we open ourselves to the challenges and joys of later life and look to developing our inner resources for managing difficult experiences, living well is possible. Throughout this book, we will draw on these opportunities for enhanced emotional regulation abilities within CAT's developmental and relational understandings over the life course to show how better health can be supported in later years. We will offer ideas for managing difficult feelings and setting realistic goals for change, as well as dealing with setbacks.

We hope that you will find the stories, ideas and strategies that follow helpful and hopeful, and that you experience first-hand that change for the better is possible.

Chapter 2: The dance of relating in later life

Elizabeth Wilde McCormick

> *'Mindful self-compassion means holding difficult emotion – fear, anger, sadness, shame and self doubt – and ourselves – in loving awareness, leading to greater ease and well-being in our daily lives.'*
>
> Chris Germer (2009, p61)

This chapter aims to first give readers a more in-depth understanding of CAT, as a relational model, and then apply its key concepts to later-life challenges through personal and professional reflections. One of the main hallmarks of CAT is its relational freedom. The model encourages each of us to develop our own form of the art of recognition. Having been involved in the development of CAT since its early days in the 1980s, I write this chapter now at the age of seventy-seven. It is an opportunity for me to reflect upon again my own learned patterns of relating, to others and to myself, and reflect upon how my awareness and understanding of them has changed as I have moved into later life. I've been asking: 'What kind of conversations am I currently having with myself and with my old, learned procedures around emotion?' I hope this chapter will offer readers an opportunity to ask the same question along with helpful insights, where change might be needed. Later life is a time to really reflect on what has been important to us but which no longer serves, and what is now really, really important and needs our time and attention.

An overview of CAT

Cognitive Analytic Therapy was developed in the early 1980s by Dr Anthony Ryle at Guy's and St Thomas' hospitals in London. It has at its heart lies the understanding that we are naturally social beings, evolving throughout our lives in a web of relationships with others. How we are in a relationship, with ourselves, with others, with ideas and life itself, plays a vital part in living a life throughout all ages and stages. The focus of CAT is to help us identify and name our own patterns of relating, to others and to ourselves, so that any unnamed, unlived emotional life may have an opportunity for healing and expression, and we are able to give ourselves more choice in our responses.

Most of our emotional responses are learned in early life. Some are helpful, such as feeling loved in relation to a loving other; feeling valued as a person just as we are, in relation to being valued by another. Other emotional patterns may be more painful and difficult, such as feeling judged and dismissed in relation to a judging or dismissing other, so we develop a conditional way of relating. For example: 'Only if I behave in a certain way will I be acceptable/loved'. CAT clearly describes these relational patterns to help us recognize our own. We also come to recognize that, having learned these emotional patterns in early life, we carry them within us, and thus will become judging of or unloving to ourselves. The resulting suffering which CAT calls core pain may be a sense of hurt, worthlessness, and hopelessness. Our core pain is unique to us, based on what, for us, was both the nature of, and our response to, the people, atmosphere and experiences of our early life. We may cope with the more negative patterns of relating by avoiding any closeness, by pleasing others but never ourselves, by using substances to drown our emotional pain, until we are able to revise this and name the learned patterns around it.

Being a highly relational therapy, CAT sets out a clear, focused programme to help us address these learned patterns of being in relationship, to oneself, to others and to the world outside, and find and practice exits if needed. We become the observer of patterns of thinking and behaving that have led to things going wrong. It is through developing a kind observer-self – the 'I' that sees 'me' – that we are able to give more space around ourselves and our reactions, to name them and also begin to understand the nature of our learned patterns of relating. This creative and unique map-making contribution of CAT helps us develop a shorthand for understanding our patterns by dividing our early learned responses into traps, dilemmas and snags. Chapter three will explore map making in more detail. CAT also helps us to name and address any unstable states of mind that confuse us and trip us up. At the heart of the work, there arises a 'window of tolerance' (Siegel, 1999), a wise space of noticing and checking, sometimes sharing; a space we benefit from cherishing. And we have this map for life, adjusting or adding or deleting it at any time. It is particularly useful for conversations in older life. We can return to the map we've made at any time and check out where we are in relation to feelings, thoughts, attitudes.

CAT began its creative process of development at Guy's and St Thomas' hospitals in London in 1983 as a brief therapy project. Dr Anthony Ryle, the founder of CAT, wanted to develop a well-developed, integrative and time-limited therapy that could be available in the NHS, and was able to be learned by different mental health professionals: doctors, psychiatrists, psychologists, nurses, social workers and many others. I was lucky enough to be part of these early days, in regular weekly creative discussions and supervision with Dr Anthony Ryle and the many other professionals who joined in the process. The Association for Cognitive Analytic Therapy is now well established with nearly fifteen hundred members in the UK, with many therapists in many different settings offering the short-term programmes of CAT. Much has been written about the work in many books. There are now therapists working with the CAT model all over the UK and beyond: in Greece, Spain, Ireland, Finland, Italy, France, Australia and New Zealand. Each country has brought their own perspectives and recognitions which are shared with us all, contributing to widening the map. The versatility of the CAT model has meant that it has been taken up by therapists offering CAT in many different settings: hospitals, day centres, with couples and young people, as well as in prisons. There are now many therapists from different therapeutic backgrounds learning and enjoying the CAT model, who have enriched CAT with music therapy, dance and art therapy, across the life span.

CAT and later life

The CAT self-help book called *Change for the Better* (McCormick, 1990) offers a clear introduction to the CAT model of relational understanding. The book has been in print since 1990 and is now in its fifth edition. I wrote the first edition in 1989, when I was forty-three. Now, I write this contribution for a new book based upon the structure of CAT with gratitude.

Conversations in Later Life is a great title for reflection upon the many different conversations we all may have as our life changes as we age, what has been let go of, and what lives on! These internal and external conversations can help us to check out where we are as we age; how many old patterns are still in operation and what, if anything, needs to be challenged. They also help to support us at a time of entering the personal unknown on the well-trodden path to aging. This also gives me the opportunity to reflect on the five different editions of *Change for the Better* with their revisions, and recognize what was influencing me at those different stages of my own life and at those times. CAT has grown alongside a general universal awareness of changing attitudes and needs, particularly towards health, towards the many different choices we now have in how and with whom we form relationships, towards fashion, and towards gender. While change may be welcome and invigorating, one of the conversations I have noticed in later life is about confusion and concern over the increasing dominance of IT, and of the relevance and place in the modern world of older generations. Also, our news is full of stories of loneliness, poverty and isolation in old age, in many different countries, as well as the divisions and heightened aggression throughout the world, different conflicts and wars, the plights of refugees, our recent pandemic.

Relational freedom is, as I have said, one of the main hallmarks of CAT, and it teaches us to recognize when we have succumbed to a trap or dilemma, or when a snag has been in operation. As we do this, we are developing and strengthening the 'eye that sees 'me''. And by pausing with our recognition from this spacious observer-self we can try something different, known as an exit in CAT. The first task is to complete the Psychotherapy File, which you will find in Appendix 1. This will help to start the process of self-reflection and understanding current struggles in the form of learned patterns of behaviour and relating, in order to consider where changes can be made. It can be helpful to keep a journal to help the process of recognizing these patterns as they arise in your daily life and any thoughts you have when completing the exercises.

Mindfulness

Part of my development and interest since 1989 has been the practice of mindfulness, which I began in 1992 after struggling to recover from meningitis. The practice of mindfulness has shown me that simply stopping, noticing the rise and fall of the breath, with acceptance, kindness and compassion, can accompany the art of recognition and observation of old patterns, and that this can make a huge difference. For example, one of my learned procedures was 'soldiering on without feeling', developed because it was not possible to sit and pause safely in my early environment. The message was 'Don't just sit there, do something'. The cost of simply sitting and noticing, even the birds and bluebells, was anger, disapproval, judgement. The bottom line would be feeling unloved, unless I pleased and fitted in. While the learned habit has had some benefits, such as getting things done, it's often pushed my body much further than she wants to go. I also learned a useful expression when I worked in the cardiac department of Charing Cross Hospital, where Dr Peter Nixon would refer to certain patients suffering from 'hurry sickness' – unable to stop, rest, or notice until their poor heart did it for them.

Since meningitis, I've learned to sit more and be still, and notice what wants to arise. Bessel van der Kolk writes that 'the body leads the way' and that 'the body does not lie' (2015). This is a great mantra for conversations with our bodies in later life. What is my body saying right now? How can I be with this kindly? As I've aged, I've also noticed that I am more anxious or afraid of ordinary things, such as getting ready to go out, remembering not to forget keys etc., and of something going wrong. I've met many people in my age bracket who, as their usual skills and confidence lessen and changes, find fear arising. Many years ago, I used to bicycle several miles from Victoria to Guy's Hospital through busy traffic, close to lorries and double-decker buses, along the Embankment and thought nothing of it. I would attend supervision and see patients, and then I would bicycle home again. I'm glad to say that I enjoyed it all and feel glad now that I did it. And I did not feel afraid then. But now, this would not be possible. Even preparing for a train or bus journey, I find myself checking everything several times. The fear is non-specific and often exaggerated. It is based upon an old belief that I must be seen to get things right and be brave, and of course to 'soldier on without feeling'. Very brave to ride a bicycle through central London! I have worked with this as time has evolved, but now, one of the conversations I have with myself is with my kind observer-self and fear. There is a mindfulness practice from the work of Thich Nhat Hanh (2012) that embraces fear and anxiety beautifully.

Exercise

- As we notice what we feel is fear or anxiety, pause, sit down if possible.
- Feel that emotion in our bodies and the accompanying thoughts such as: 'I must, I should, but I can't and I am hopeless…' etc.
- So, we simply notice and stop.
- We say: 'Hello, Fear, my friend. I know you are there and I'm there for you.'
- We befriend those fearful aspects that possibly have never been named and kindly held.

Developmental understanding

The understanding behind the structure of CAT is that we come into life with our own unique self and are a bit like a seed planted into the garden of life. This unique seed carries the essence of who we are as well as the genes connected to our biological relatives. But we all must adjust to the environment into which we are born, which means that some of us must bend and twist a long way from our original seed in order to survive. Very few people get exactly the right soil for their growth. But all of us have good survival skills and we adapt. The structure of CAT offers a clear way of naming and mapping our learned survival habits, and identifying them as traps, dilemmas and snags. Each one is accompanied by patterns of thinking, feeling and relationship, to oneself and to others. CAT helps us to find creative ways to name the patterns of response we have taken for granted, and to develop realistic goals for the process of change if change is needed. We can find resources to help us in the process of realization and changing, and we can clear the ground of unhelpful learned patterns or old beliefs. One of the useful conversations we can have in later life, when it can feel as if there's not much time left, is to reflect on some of our old patterns, as outlined below, and ask ourselves if they are still active and if anything needs to change. One of my early teachers said: 'It's never too late to have a happy childhood!' As we reflect and begin a dialogue internally, we can use the time to feel more real, more present and closer to our original seed with which we came into life. It's never too late...

The dance of relating

Everything we experience about being a person happens in context with 'others'. We awaken first through our bodies and our awareness of smell, touch, feel and sound. This can be sensed as pleasant or unpleasant, good, bad, loud, soft, nice or nasty. The reciprocal nature of relating with others begins early in our experiences with caregivers as we come slowly into consciousness and begin to gain a sense of our environment and who we are within it. The experience of being held lovingly and safely helps us create an internalized healthy island of feeling secure and loved. We are also able to give and receive love. An experience of being abandoned or neglected leads to the development of an abandoning in relation to abandoned sense of self, with feelings of being dropped or unwanted and therefore believing we must be unlovable, even bad. All of us carry a mixed repertoire of reciprocal patterns learned from early relating. They can be reflected upon at any time so that adjustments may be made to the more problematic procedures.

It's not just *what* happens to us, but what we *make of what* happens to us. In later life, as we begin reflecting more on our learned patterns of relating, we can offer ourselves an overview of our own development of relating, inner and outer, with ourselves and with others. We can see, perhaps more clearly in our maturity, which learned patterns are still active and whether they are helpful or unhelpful. The following is a table of patterns that may have dominated our relationships. We may be aware of most of them, but they are worth looking through before we name our own traps, dilemmas and snags. If you haven't already completed the Psychotherapy File (Appendix 1) maybe try before reading on further.

The following chart is included in the fifth edition of *Change for the Better* (McCormick, 2017) – perhaps read these and see if any resonate with you.

Table 2.1 Patterns of care that can dominate our relationships until we revise them

The way we experienced care	What we felt	Attempted solution (survival pattern)	Recipricol role (with self and others)
ABSENT Rejecting Abandoning	rejected abandoned	placating parental child	rejecting ↔ rejected abandoning ↔ abandoned
CONDITIONAL Judging Belittling Demanding Blaming	judged humiliated crushed blamed	striving striving hypervigilance hypervigilance	judging ↔ judged admiring ↔ rubbished exacting ↔ crushed blaming ↔ blamed
TOO TIGHT Overcontrolling Fused dependency Flattening	restricted merged flattened	rebellion flight into fantasy giving in	controlling ↔ controlled merging ↔ merged flattening ↔ flattened
TOO LOOSE Anxious Not there Abandoning	anxious fragile abandoned	avoidance anxious striving 'nowhere world'	abandoning ↔ abandoned conditional /disapproving distancing ↔ distanced
TOO BUSY Overlooking Depriving Silencing	overlooked deprived silenced	excessive striving searching 'not there'	overlooking ↔ overlooked depriving ↔ deprived silencing ↔ silenced
ENVIOUS Envious Hated Picking	envied hated picked on	magical guilt self-sabotage self-harm	harming ↔ harmed hating ↔ hated picking ↔ picked on
NEGLECTING Neglecting Physical neglect Emotional neglect Mental neglect Attacking	neglecting hurt hurt/angry fragmented attacked	can't take care mood swings feel in bits unstable states develop 'false' self	neglecting ↔ neglected switching states unstable states unstable states attacking ↔ attacked →

The way we experienced care	What we felt	Attempted solution (survival pattern)	Recipricol role (with self and others)
ABUSIVE Abusing	abused	bully/victim	abusing ↔ abused fantasy of perfect care
VIOLENT Abusing states	hurt/abused	split into fragments unexpressed rage	fragmented hitting out ↔ hitting self

Exercise

Self to self

- Rest your attention on the general flavour of your close relationships, starting with the relationship you have via inner dialogue with yourself.
- Take your time. Notice how you think about and speak to yourself inside.
- You may find you have imaginary conversations, with real-life or fictional others, and that there are themes to these.
- Themes might include trying to be heroic, or happy, or pleasing someone; conversations may be being critical, judging or encouraging, hopeful or longing toward an imaginary other.

Self to other

- Notice how you anticipate how others will behave toward you, especially in close relationships.
- Notice how this anticipation manifests in the tension in your body, in your thoughts.
- You may anticipate and hope for special words only to be met with words that do not meet your hopes and expectations and you end up feeling disappointed or dashed.
- You may anticipate harshness, criticism and hold yourself back or even make yourself vulnerable to what is expected.
- Notice all your reactions when with others.
- As you explore your own reciprocal roles and notice the core pain of the child derived role such as punished, criticized, bullied, forgotten, think about what you would feel if you saw a child being treated as you were.

Traps, dilemmas and snags in later life

Traps

Certain kinds of thinking and acting result in a 'vicious circle' when, however hard we try, things seem to get worse rather than better. CAT describes the following traps:

'Doing what others want, or placation trap'

We might have learned to keep ourselves safe from judgement or criticism by trying to please others, do whatever they want and try to keep the peace. But we end up being used and feeling abused, taken for granted, and our uncertainty about ourselves, particularly our self-worth, grows. As long as we are using all our energy trying to please others we are unable to develop a real sense of ourselves, what we might like, the voice we need to develop in order to be ourselves.

Martha became aware of how much this learned trap of placation was still affecting her life during her early sixties. She developed rheumatoid arthritis and felt unwell a lot of the time. She also found asking for help from her partner and children very difficult. Her old belief was that she should manage and should not make trouble for anyone. She felt out of control if she were not pleasing others and feared both ridicule and rejection. She spoke of postponing asking for help saying to herself, 'I'll manage – I'll be better tomorrow'. She feared the helplessness she had seen in other people her age and carried a lot of fear and anxiety. Eventually, she had a bad fall and was admitted to hospital. Her feet were swollen and bleeding and she had bandaged them up as best she could. Suddenly, there she was in a place she had feared for so long, helpless, vulnerable, exposed and full of fear. Her 30-year-old son sat by her bedside many times, bringing her fruit and magazines. He held her hand kindly and said, 'Mum, why did you not tell us you needed help?' When she looked tearful, he said gently 'You've always been there for us and helped us. It's our turn to help you now. Please accept.'

These words melted her heart, and this was the beginning of a transformation of a pattern that had been dominant: 'Unless I am doing what others want, pleasing, being useful and in charge, I will be rejected, unloved, shoved out, and I will feel empty and worthless.'

The changes didn't occur overnight, but she began to practice noticing, making a space for stopping and revising the old belief, and then taking the risk of sometimes saying 'no'. She recognized that the old belief was based upon her early life and her mother's voice: 'Don't think anyone's going to be interested in your ideas or feelings. Just get on with making sure you put others first.' She recognized the child in her that held these beliefs and was still dominating her even though she was now over sixty. She also learned to listen to what was happening with her body: shoulders tight, mouth down, head down… When we met, I watched her eyes brighten, she no longer walked with her head down, she looked me in the eye. All this contributed to a growth in strength that changed her life in a positive way.

Depressed thinking trap

Thinking about ourselves in a depressed way can become a habit. For example, we may have thoughts such as 'I'm bound to do this badly', or we might expect ourselves to be doomed in some way. This sort of thinking can build up so that we feel depressed about ourselves. It's the thinking itself that develops into a trap when it becomes habitual. We may not be aware that we are thinking in a depressed way as we take it for granted, as if it's just how things are. We may even think there's no point in trying to change anything. What we can do is to monitor our negative thoughts for a week and then stop and try to see where they stem from. Write them down and then reflect. We may find patterns such as, 'I'm not going into that place, they don't even see me; I'll just stay here and watch television; there's no point doing anything else…'

One of the conversations we may begin to have in later life is: 'Why am I so down on everything? Why do I feel so unwelcome, so doomed? Why do I no longer feel adventurous, excited, happy and prepared to be challenged by learning something new? Is it all down to my age?' It's as if we believe that growing older makes us less interesting, less competent, even a nuisance. This trap, as well as the placation trap, can become more prevalent in later life, particularly if we are retired or suffering loss and are alone a lot. We need to develop a kindly and encouraging internal voice that inspires us to seek others who respond to us kindly and find others happy to bring us out of the trap.

Social isolation trap

Sometimes we may think 'I'm better off on my own', particularly if we have become unfamiliar with meeting new people. If we've held down a busy job that has taken all our energy, we may have to develop new skills with people we don't know or people we know but haven't become as involved with as we might be. If we've found it too difficult to be around others socially, we may get into the habit of just being on our own. If we've grown up in an environment where everyone was busy, we may not have learned any social skills. Sometimes in later life this trap may be triggered following bereavement. I remember on one of the early occasions I braved going out following my husband's death in 1999, I was with a group of people and became tearful. Someone noticed and said 'Oh, haven't you got over it yet?' Another person moved forward and put her arm around me. So, I had these two opposite responses. If this had been one of my procedures I might have concentrated on the former and not allowed myself to be nourished by the latter, maintaining my isolation and negative self-belief.

Avoidance trap

We learn to avoid when whatever it is that we are avoiding feels too difficult. This might be in relation to others, to tasks, to future planning, or anything that just feels too difficult. It's useful to reflect upon and make a list of things we have avoided over the years, and which might have built up into a habit. As a way of managing conflict, we learn to avoid difficulty on any level, which means we don't develop the skill of managing. It means that if we need to change this, we must be brave!

Exercise

Reflect and list anything that you think you have avoided over the years, perhaps to keep the peace or because you worried that you could not have coped. Does avoidance serve you well in terms of living the life you want?

Recently, I was in Norfolk with some old, wonderful friends. We were walking along the huge sandy beaches with our dogs, admiring the oystercatchers. As we stepped away from the beach, we encountered sand dunes. My fit friends happily ascended them and ran down the daunting slopes, but I found it really difficult, especially going down. My friend David, a retired GP, took me by the arm and guided me kindly. As we came to the flat sands he said, thoughtfully, 'Liz, now you live in a bungalow do you go upstairs?'

'Oh no, I don't have to do that now', I answered.

And he said, again kindly, 'But if you're not doing stairs anymore, you might be getting bungalow knees.'

This is what he called them when in GP practice. Very clear and expressive. I was shocked, and there was a time when I might have felt chastised for my avoidance, and I might have chastised myself. But his kindness and explanation – that he had come across many patients with these knees – made it 'ordinary', which encouraged me to use stairs every day. I have, happily and gladly, after receiving his kindness, been putting it into operation and it has got easier, and I've expressed my gratitude. One of the later-in-life conversations has a lot to do with the body, living in an aging body and avoiding anything tricky or which hurts.

Low self-esteem

This becomes a trap when we continually compare ourselves with others and find ourselves wanting. We find ourselves in a reciprocal role of judging in relation to judged and found wanting. The tendency is to compare ourselves with people who are stars, who are brilliant, rather than notice what we naturally do well. This can become a habit we take for granted until we stop and revise it. Low self-esteem may also become more accentuated as we age and realize we cannot accomplish what we used to and are unable to find alternatives. We can lament lost opportunities or feel regret for paths not followed. We can also reflect on what was happening then, how we were feeling at those times. Was it connected to our concern for others or feeling we did not have enough courage?

Exercise

Reflect upon all the things you have done well – you could ask a friend you trust to help if this feels too difficult to do yourself. Next, write a list of all the things you realize now that you have done well, especially when you consider what was going on at the time. Keep it with you to look at every day.

There is a saying, 'better late than never' – so why not try now, in later life, some of the things you've avoided or feared you wouldn't be able to accomplish? Even if it's just meeting new people or experimenting with new ideas and events – music, walking, travelling, conversations.

Fear of hurting others trap

This trap may be developed in our early life when there is a fear of strong emotions such as anger within families, and we learn to believe that, if we are angry, it will be harmful, especially to those on whom we depend. We may also feel that we will be punished. Sometimes, strict parenting or schooling may leave us feeling that it's impossible to express what we really feel or need, so it's very hard for us to be free to be assertive in any form. But we all feel anger and frustration; it's an appropriate response at times, and it's important that we find useful ways of expressing it. Bottling it up, letting it fester, can cause us harm, especially if it's long term. Turning our anger against ourselves is often the root of self-punishing acts such as self-deprivation, eating disorders, and actual self-harm, as clearly illustrated in Paul's personal account in Chapter 6. We may also unconsciously seek out partners with whom we cannot express what we feel, positive or negative, but feel under their control. All because this is what we have learned and expect.

It's helpful to spend a bit of time reflecting on how we have carried anger, and when we have been able to recognize that is what we feel. I have a lovely story from one woman who had been widowed for five years and met another man. They started seeing each other and each Friday he would come home from work and they would have a meal together. One Friday, he was in the sitting room and it was her turn to prepare the meal. She was something of a perfectionist – often the way we manage fears of hurting others – and really wanted this new man to be impressed. When she took a dish out of the oven it had been overcooked and she felt so disappointed she kicked the oven and shouted, thinking that he could not hear. But the man ran in and got hold of her and said, 'Yes, yes, you be angry, it's all OK'. They hugged and laughed together. She learned that he was totally comfortable with anger, his own and others', and, expressing it in a useful way, he did not hold onto it or resent her if she became angry. It was a new and positive experience for her as she was moving into her late sixties.

Dilemmas

Dilemmas arise when we feel as though our choices as to how to be and act are divided into bleak opposites. We choose the pole of the dilemma that is most comfortable for our survival self, usually because we see the alternative as much worse. The result is a kind of psychological lopsidedness which we act on without thinking. For example: either I keep feelings bottled up or I risk making a mess. There is no middle way, or 'good enough' here. We never learn to find the full landscape of our own feelings. It's good to reflect on what a 'mess' might be for us. What sort of feelings do we consider messy? Our bodies can lead the way here, notice what our body does when we say the word 'mess' in relation to feeling. Is it crying, being angry and showing it? Is it connected to neediness? It's possible that, in later life, we do in fact experience ourselves as more needy than we would like, and we might even work hard to keep things tightly bottled up. Where did we learn that some feelings are messy and to be avoided? Those of us brought up with Victorian values may well have learned to keep a tight bodice and corset over our stronger feelings, as if they were in some way repulsive or too self-exposing. But in later life, we need to look carefully at what the cost of keeping feelings under wraps could be.

Exercise

Ask yourself:

- Which feelings do you bottle up and why?
- When and where did you learn to do this?
- It may have been an important part of your survival in earlier life, but is it useful now?

It does seem that we need to find ways to express all our feelings as we get older, otherwise we enter a dry and difficult path of isolation. And it can feel really good to simply let go of them!

Perfect or guilty dilemma

This dilemma is dominated by the need for perfection. We may strive to meet impossible self-imposed standards but end up never feeling good enough. And if we are not striving, we feel guilty and sometimes empty and lost. It's as if we have learned to become slaves to a system of perfection imposed upon us. It's as if this is the only way to feel emotionally and physically safe. There can be burnout associated with this dilemma and, if it is not questioned, we may develop an obsessional habit and always feel empty inside. When I have named this need for perfection and asked people if it is their choice, they often look puzzled. It's as if there is absolutely no choice. Again, this is back to survival. In her book

Will I Ever Be Good Enough, Karyl McBride (2008) writes about the burden of striving to please mothers for whom nothing is ever good enough and the tendency to strive for perfection in order to attempt to gain love.

Given a choice, most of us wish to enter later life with peace of mind and learn to be comfortable with doing our best whatever the result. But with this dilemma it seems that finding what enough is, or 'good enough' looks like, has not been a choice we've ever felt we could have. And whatever the high achievements we have made, it can feel as if it is never enough to satisfy the emptiness inside.

Perfect control or perfect mess dilemma

This dilemma is related to any experience we may have had with anything that felt 'messy' in our early life and which we felt we had to control out of fear of reprimand or punishment. The mess may be related to spilt milk, to untidiness, to body functions or to feelings, especially ones that seem to explode out of us, from shouting, screaming or weeping loudly, to stomach rumbles and farts, anything that seems out of control. If we learn that mess of any kind is bad and likely to earn us punishment, we feel we must learn methods of control such as tidying, cleaning and sweeping. We may limit what we do freely only to our safe comfort zones, never daring to take a risk with anything new.

One of the conversations in later life needs to include our finding a sense of reasonable and manageable control and safety without reprimand. For growing older always brings certain messes and challenges in both body and mind. We may not be able to continue with our control rituals but instead find creative ways to accept our struggling bodies with real kindness.

Greedy or self-punishing dilemma

This dilemma finds expression in patterns such as gambling, eating disorders such as bulimia, or compulsively buying things we do not need only to have to keep returning them. The origins of the dilemma are related to our basic needs which have been unmet completely or have become compromised. It's as if we must ration all our desires, as if they were forbidden. We can only allow ourselves something for a short time during which we have to eat/buy/gamble as much as possible. There may be just a moment of satisfaction after which guilt takes over and then we have to make up for it by punishing ourselves. There is a deep sadness to this dilemma. Anita, in her therapy, said: 'I feel so sad for all those painful years of bingeing and starving, sad for the lost soul I was then. I feel so sad for the young woman I was who might have enjoyed a freer time in her twenties. But I am so glad I was able to have it recognized now through therapy. I can now listen more carefully when any appetite threaten to sweep me away. I have learned what enough is. So lucky.'

Busy carer or empty loner

Loneliness and the fear of loneliness are prevalent as we get older. The children are gone, and we are with what is often called an 'empty nest'. Perhaps we have not had the opportunity to have children, and this is a regret for us. We may find ourselves alone, unexpectedly. We may have retired reluctantly or been forced to retire early (retirement will be explored further in Chapter 5). Whatever the external event that has triggered this dilemma for us, it's a challenge to sit with feelings of emptiness and our fear of it. We may try and fill it with all kinds of activities until we can stop and ask ourselves: what do I really want now? What do I really need? What part of me needs nourishment? What activity, what company would I describe as the most nourishing in the last week?

Another question may be: has being a carer for others meant that we have not given ourselves time to consider our own needs? Has our 'need to be needed' dominated our relationships and our lives. Has it brought us satisfaction and happiness? If so, it's important to rejoice in this and at the same time consider how to recognize our own needs right now, and what sort of care for ourselves we might need as we age. There may be dreams, activities or hobbies we've had to put on hold because others' needs were more important. 'I'll do it later – there's not enough time for that now…' We'll explore these themes further in Chapter 7.

That question we come back to as we sit down with our well-learned habits and patterns of thinking is: 'What do I most need right now?'

Exercise

- Having read through the CAT description of traps and dilemmas, which procedures dominate you?
- Let us spend a few moments reflecting on your current judgements of yourself.
- Whose voices do you hear? Your own, as it is now, or a much younger voice? A parental or authoritative voice? If it is not your own voice, whose is it?

Snags and self-sabotage – 'Yes… but…'

Self-sabotage occurs when we avoid pleasure or success. Or, if we are successful and happy, 'we feel as if we have to pay in some way for our pleasure or success. We may tell ourselves that we could go on that exotic holiday but… Or perhaps we have achieved that important interview but do not turn up for it. We may immediately put on the weight we've lost. It's as if we cannot allow ourselves to receive anything good. The sabotage may be a force within us that is deeply woven and hidden, subconscious, or a force embedded in society like a glass ceiling or a taboo.

Magical guilt and envy

It's very difficult to feel envious and recognize it, and it's very difficult to be on the receiving end of envy. Being actively envied by others, especially within your own family, can cause you to feel bad about something you have - good looks, talent, love even - which the other person feels they lack. It can lead you to neglect some aspects of yourself and feel bad about your gifts. Arranging unconsciously to operate a snag or self-sabotage may occur because you've been envied by a close family member and experienced it as an attack.

Guilt, then, becomes 'magical', because it is guilt for something you cannot possibly be guilty of. It is not a conscious thought, but an unconscious process and it can dominate your actions or non-actions.

It tends to develop in early life unconsciously, before we can assess what is happening, and we take 'magical' responsibility for things going wrong in the family. If we are kept in the dark about the reality of what is happening and people all around us are cross or upset, our omnipotent child's fear can be that it must be something we have done and therefore our fault. If a family member suffered from an illness or depression, or there was a death in the family, and this is not discussed so that we are relieved of the burden of worrying that it is our fault, we can feel guilty. The result in adult life is the false belief that, if we have something good or are happy or successful, 'it must be at someone else's expense. We pay for it by not enjoying or celebrating our own skills or aptitudes.

This was brought home to me very profoundly by someone I saw many years ago who was a professional singer. Alice had a beautiful voice and had been celebrated on the concert circuit. But as she became more successful, she developed a pattern of not turning up for interviews, thus sabotaging her opportunities. She sought help when she realized things had gone too far and she had stopped singing, was just eking out a living giving a few lessons here and there and living alone in a small flat with very little income. She had had a sister who died young, before Alice was born and her mother never got over it. Alice remembered her mother speaking wistfully of this sister and she felt that her mother was resentful of her for being alive when her sister was dead . Alice had a sense that she was in some way responsible for her mother's unhappiness, because she was not the earlier child. An altogether impossible burden. In addition to this, her mother often showed signs of envying Alice, for being alive and free enough to make a go of her natural talents when her mother or her dead sister could not. 'It's alright for you...' her mother would often say.

It was her magical guilt that was behind her withdrawal from her singing career. A desperate attempt to get away from crippling feelings of guilt and heaviness. Slowly, she began to understand and take stock, and take the risk of beginning again with her musical career. Eventually, and wonderfully, she began to sing again, to allow herself to enjoy her talents and celebrate them. She even invited her mother to celebrate with her as they were lucky enough to still be alive. She could sing in memory of her dead sister.

If I must, then I won't. If I must not, then I will

This dilemma is a feisty response to restriction! It is built upon the pain of a sense of restricted self and as if the only way out is resistance. It's as if 'the proof of my existence is my resistance'. It may have developed early in life as we felt our natural freedoms to be curtailed. We may have had many freedoms early on, to play as we wished, express ourselves through different mediums, share and speak on all levels, and then it is suddenly taken away from us. I have met several men – as well as a few women – who were sent to boarding school early, at seven or eight, which many feel now is almost criminal, and who developed this dilemma. One man, now in his seventies, had recently undergone an operation for lung cancer. He had been always a rebel, but has managed to hold down a good job as a builder and enjoyed a full family life. One of his pleasures, now seen as naughty these days, was smoking. Not only did he enjoy the sensation, but it was a time when he could be alone and feel free of demands or of having to respond. He described one interview with his consultant and a senior lung cancer nurse. They were discussing his smoking habits which he had reduced hugely since his diagnosis, from ten each day to five. As the nurse was about to pass him a leaflet about counselling for giving up smoking, the consultant stepped in and suggested the following: 'Why not just have a few puffs each day? You can enjoy this.' He spoke as if from one conspirator to another. But the result was startling. This man did as the consultant suggested, cut down to one cigarette each day from which he enjoyed three or four puffs three times each day, after breakfast, lunch and supper.

The stubbornness within this dilemma can cause real difficulty in a close relationship unless it is recognized and respected and ways found, like the wise consultant, to offer a manageable way forward.

Changing and aging challenges

Having outlined the patterns involved in the CAT structure of traps, dilemmas and snags, it's helpful to reflect on the following areas of concern that can be prevalent as we get older. We can then allow them to become part of our conversations in later life as we notice which traps, dilemmas or snags are still with us, and what steps we have taken already, or could take, to relate to them more helpfully.

Everything changes every day; this is the only certainty we have. Whether we see them or not, throughout our lives we have opportunities for change, and, of course, some changes are thrust upon us. Aging is inevitable for us all, but many of us find that we have made little preparation. A map is always vital when we are in a new country or approaching a new area. Every stage of the aging process is always a new country, and while the map is not the country, it indicates what we might come across. Brambles, rivers, barren fields, mountains, wild beasts... But there may also be some territory where kindness and helpfulness reside, which has been previously unknown or forgotten; which is waiting for our attention and return. Knowing our learned patterns and developing a compassionate observer in the 'I' that sees 'me' can help us to revise whatever is required as we are challenged by the natural process of aging.

Exercise

- I have reflected on the many conversations I have had in my later life with others on the same path. To follow Tony Ryle's lead, I asked myself and others the following questions:
- What is now most important to you, and what is not important?
- What conversations am I having with myself, consciously and unconsciously?
- Through whose eyes do I look at myself at different times?

Loss and emptiness: old and new

Aging always involves loss, and the emptiness and sadness that can follow an experience of loss. There are obvious losses in later life such as: 'the empty nest', where we miss the company and structure of children and feeling part of a new life growing. This is especially so if we carry a procedure of 'needing to be needed' to help our own identity or as a way of giving our life meaning.

We may have retired and miss our work and all the structures that went with having a job, however small. Sometimes this is unexpected, and it takes time to make the necessary adjustments.

We may have had to move home. When this is not our choice there is a huge adjustment and a loss of the familiar surroundings we may have known for years.

We may have been diagnosed and are learning to live with poor eyesight or memory, a debilitating physical condition such as arthritis, or more serious, such as MS. Our response to these conditions is, of course, always individual, and the help and support we receive are vital. But how are we, internally, in response? Do we allow ourselves to take the time to mourn fully, whatever we have lost? Are we able to face disappointment or frailty? Are we able to ask for help? We inevitably touch different forms of loss as we age, and the procedures we've learned to cope with them may dominate our responses. Do we feel we have to find replacements, to fill any gaps, to work harder on some project? And if we don't do this, do we feel as if we've failed? Do we judge ourselves harshly? I've heard several people say 'Don't let yourself grow old, Liz', and asked them what they meant. I've asked: what sort of 'old' do you feel is unacceptable? Do you mean old and therefore cranky? There is usually a laugh and a shrug, and the inference is that somehow growing older is giving up. Listening to one's own body, mind and heart is not giving up, it's designing new paths. And it doesn't happen overnight! These are conversations we all need to be having in later life to carve out the shape we most need for the being we are. Self-judgement that makes us push on regardless or because we feel we 'ought' to is not useful. These issues related to loss and endings will be explored further in Chapter 8.

The body calls, and often leads the way

The challenge here is how to be with an aging body helpfully. Perhaps the answer is to ask more open questions and see what happens, rather than judging it as useless because it isn't now what it once was, or pushing it to be younger. 'Dear body, you've seen me through years and years, thank you! What do you most need now in later life?' Our bodies do tell us if we listen. I have an example to illustrate this. While recovering from meningitis, which took a very long time, I sat down one morning to meditate and I said to myself, rather crossly: 'If only I could feel well!' I then heard a voice inside say clearly: 'And what would you do with your wellness?' I was both shocked and moved by this because I knew then that I would probably try to get into the fast lane again. I was in my late forties and led an extremely busy working and personal life. But this response from inside my own body and self was startling and moving, and helpful. I began listening more attentively and letting my body be a guide. Other people have told me that, when they listen, the answer comes. Reconnect with the exercise in Chapter 1, sitting quietly and noticing what arises. Try to integrate this into your daily routine. Our bodies might also be saying please make sure you do the exercises so that your joints and muscles are kept in circulation.

There can be a temptation to try to ignore our bodies as we get older, and sometimes it's not until something happens to us physically that we really stop and take notice. We must revise procedures that demand more of us than is appropriate and require us to take a new attitude. We may find our body has been calling for us to slow down and sometimes to stop, rather than waiting for ill-health ''to force the issue. More chronic difficulties, such as arthritis, mean that we have to go much more slowly and spend time exercising and regulating our body's efforts. In being forced to slow down by our bodies, we may have to enter the 'core pain' of CAT such as feeling worthless or empty, which can be painful. Again, as we realize our internal emotional suffering, we have the opportunity to say 'Hello, my friend, I know you are there. I will be with you positively.'

To give another example from my work in the cardiac department of Charing Cross Hospital in the 1980s, I was at a multi-disciplinary meeting of professionals caring for a recent heart attack patient. He was young, at forty-three, and he had been admitted to the ward following a second heart attack. Sadly, he had died on the ward. One of the occupational therapists who had been looking after him described him as someone 'who thought he could run past death itself…' I found this very profound, and it was sad that he had not been given the time to adjust his attitude to living in a precious body.

There can also be a tendency to take a lot of medication in later life, which may be helpful, indeed vital, but if it is accompanied by not listening to the language of our bodies it is simply bypassing what we could learn.

> Another client, Freda said:
>
> 'I am learning to sit with my painful hands and the difficulty I have doing basic things such as gardening, cooking, even getting dressed sometimes. And when I sit and look at my hands, many difficult feelings arise. Sometimes I cry. It's not because I feel sorry for myself but it's so awful to feel empty and useless and constantly having to ask for help. There's also the pull of 'hurry sickness', which I learned early on from the voices from the past who say 'Don't just sit there do something.' But if I remember my healthy island, where I notice and recognize, I can sit with these old voices in simple recognition and not judge them. Then it's more possible to find some compassion, to remember again the kind voices that have been around recently in my therapy and my reading group and to bring them inside. To find a kind voice that says to my hands 'I will look after you so you can do what's possible', and that's kind to those awful feelings: 'It's OK to be just where you are whatever you are feeling'.'

This is when our observer-self becomes a compassionate observer, offering us a kindness that we can learn and practice. We'll explore compassion and acceptance more in Chapter 4.

Success and gains

My late husband used to say, 'If you can only have it good once in your life, have it good at the end!' He was half joking, but I am beginning to understand something of what he meant. Later life is a time to really reflect what has been important, but which no longer serves, and what is now important and needs our time and attention. We may find that we now have the time to give attention to an interest we've always had, a hobby or a love that we've never had time to develop before, or which we've never taken seriously. It's a time to find a real acceptance of the life we've had so far, whatever it has brought us into, and to find ways to feel and say that we did our best with what we were given. That is all any of us can ask for. We all know artists and writers who continue creating successfully into their nineties, such as PD James and David Hockney, and many people only discover their talents when they have time to develop them or have found unexpected happiness in later life through meeting someone special who becomes a friend or partner.

Regret and forgiveness

As we experience time running out for us, our thoughts often lead us to reflect on the past, on all experiences, both positive and negative. As explored in Chapter 1, there is often a natural developmental shift towards life review in older age. There may be missed opportunities, things that have gone wrong, paths not travelled. What do we notice about the tone of our thoughts on this? Do we judge ourselves and feel guilty? When we can come alongside the events in the past that have caused us pain we can reflect, write or share them so that our conversations open out from inside us. In doing so, we may find gaps and questions we have not yet pondered as we consider the person we were at the time of regret. There may be some important grieving to be done, grieving for what has been lost internally or externally, and then stepping into the possibility of forgiveness. Forgiveness of oneself is an important and profound experience in later life. In her beautiful book *Forgiveness*, Marina Cantacuzino (2022, p118) writes that we can 'use the emotion of remorse creatively so that it becomes a creative force'.

Worry

Many people describe feeling more 'thin on the ground' in later life. Worry, anxiety, even catastrophizing, can be part of our inner conversations as we grow older and dampen enjoyment or relaxation.

This is especially true of worry that is repetitive and irrational. Worry for things that have not happened or are unlikely to happen. It's as if we've suddenly become thinner-skinned. So many basic tasks seem to take longer, or we find them more difficult. It feels important to include conversations with our worries that we write down or take for a walk. We can listen rather than act immediately, and we can be kind. In taking our worries for a walk, we invite them to look out every now and then, for the birds, and the growing plants. This can help us to become more open to our senses. What can we see, feel, smell, hear? It's about being, not doing, not acting on irrational worry, only if our worry has a practical reality. Notice all the times when you don't worry, how has that happened?

Enjoyment and meaning

While we may regret missed opportunities, there are always new ones if we remain open. The process of aging is greatly supported by remaining open, even to things we once said we'd never do! There may be activities we had to give up when we were younger such as singing, piano playing, a reading group, a sewing group. It's never too late to take lessons if we have become rusty over time. Some villages and small towns have community shared activities at which people can get together to make or mend things, take along repairs, sew new garments, go on group walks, learn bridge or take up ballroom dancing. All good for concentration! Noticing where we most experience pleasure and enjoyment can feel new. Finding self-acceptance with new experiences and not judging them as being old-fogeyish is important and energy giving.

Summary

CAT offers us an understanding from which we can name and change problematic patterns that have kept a hold on us throughout our lives. Just as important is to value the things we have done and feel good about them. I hope this chapter has offered readers an opportunity to develop new insights into relational patterns, both what has been important but also what can be let go of, along with what matters now and that needs more time and attention. To be working at making changes and living a better life, despite one's advancing years, is both brave and possible.

Chapter 3: Mapping a lifetime of stories

Steve Potter

Introduction

This chapter is a guide to having conversations in later life that are helped by making word maps with pen and paper to spontaneously track and guide what we discuss. It takes us to the heart of Cognitive Analytic Therapy (CAT) and to the heart of what it feels like to talk deeply and genuinely about ourselves and our world in the later stages of life.

The chapter starts by establishing a distinction between *telling a personal story* (the events, drama and people of a unique memory or experience) and *finding a narrative* (the story about the story, its message, the truth we draw from it or that has been imposed on it). Narratives explain, justify or reveal what the story is about. In therapy, we don't start with the narrative, and we don't jump to conclusions about the narrative, but let the story breathe and tell us something new. If we think we know what the story is about too quickly (oh, it is about an old man) we may bypass the unscripted and spontaneous moments of discovering new feelings, new narratives or fragments of old and hidden ones.

If I tell you I am from the Baby Boomer generation, I am giving you the narrative before the lived experience of the story. If I tell you of memories of the rationing of eggs and chocolate, and that the only fruit available was seasonal from the nearby orchards of the 1950s, or dancing the twist in the local youth club to the first Beatles hit, 'Twist and Shout', in 1962, then I am inviting you and me into a hotchpotch of stories partly just to celebrate and relive them but also to ask what all that was about as we search for the narratives and test and retest their authority, and relive and discover them from the inside of each remembered story.

Narratives are sometimes so apparent that we barely get the story underway before its meaning breaks in and the telling is done (see the example later of Jimmy the grumpy old so-and-so). Stories don't always have narratives. They can just be told for the joy and drama or emotional catharsis of the shared telling and the freedom of the voicing – as in, I don't know what to make of this, but I feel better for the saying of it with someone. However, mostly, we have a deep need for narrative coherence and to bring the stories of our memories and experiences home to a meaningful and familiar conclusion.

As I see it, CAT does something simple, flexible and remarkable by making a distinction between stories and narratives. It offers the tools to map out the patterns of relating that link and separate personal stories and social narratives. I have learned that mapping out our words as we talk about ourselves can help us stay openly in between the local stories of our lives with all their hidden treasures and the general narratives that have carried us along for better or worse. The words and markings on paper become tools that bring the conversation out and create a triangle between memory, the retelling in the moment and what we are searching to say. We can free the story from a fixed narrative or open our eyes to the interplay between several narratives in one story. Indeed, what we are searching for in therapy is narrative freedom, where we can wander in and out of the stories of our own and other people's lives and not be tied to one story but, on the contrary, feel a certain sense of being our own creative first-time authors together in those moments. It offers a chance to discover a renewed authorship to our lives as we unravel the personal from the social and the past from the present.

Let me delve into an example from my childhood memories, where a collection of toy figures was the tool that helped me have the conversations I needed at the time. I can tell you stories of playing what was then called 'cowboys and Indians' (finger-sized plastic figurines in various postures) in my 1950s childhood. From them, looking back, I could draw out narratives of gender, empire and racism, of working-class whiteness, inferiority, bravery and loyalty that framed my formative years. I could not see or name the narratives at the time, but I lived and breathed them and soaked them into my view of the world as I played with the toys to make up my own stories. But not entirely. These plastic toy figures were all male stereotypes, and mostly warlike, carrying rifles, bows and tomahawks. Over the primary years of six to nine (no doubt men of my age will remember their own versions of this), I had accumulated eight cowboys and eight Indians, and they interacted under my guidance on the living room carpet, alternately hiding behind chair legs or underneath threadbare bits of the carpet. I had my favourites: Lasso Larry, whose raised arms were poised with rope to catch a steer, and Chief Sitting Bull, who stood serene, with folded arms and full-feathered headdress. I had a relationship with them individually and as a collective which resisted the simple binary and racist split between cowboys and Indians. I gave them relationships with each other, which were not set by the expected stereotypes but driven more by me projecting my childhood needs into them.

In hindsight, I see that these toys were essential and formative conversational aids, and they helped me shape my own stories in and out of the dominant narratives. They were individually brave, shy, foolish or silent; some were more feminine and chatty, others more tight-lipped and male. They were the assistants to mixed feelings, my friends, who helped me find a voice and an inner dialogue but they also colonized my imagination. They were the stand-in actors or puppets of all that was going on around me in the world of the early 1950s. With those miniature toys, I learned a lesson that still holds good for me, which is that it helps to have tools and props to facilitate a conversation and find multiple voices. Pen and paper have replaced the toy figures as my conversational aid and projective space. We can and do refuse old narratives and choose new ones in the later years of life. I want to show how CAT and its mapping and writing tools and skills can help.

This chapter has fictionalized examples of narratives mapped out from stories and conversations using CAT mapping tools of reciprocal emotionally charged roles and procedures (the workings and use of which will be explained). Jane's *triple whammy* combination of a trapped way of thinking, binary either/or choices of behaviour and a self-forbidding snag. Jimmy has a pattern (narrative) of *grumpiness* through which he sees himself and his world and he justifies the grumpiness as an inevitable feature of later life. For Mary, there is the important need for *happy dreams* and her 'Australia' dream as an aid to daily reality, and for Bihar there is *the empathy trap* that can catch her, and all of us, unexpectedly at times, when faced with the emotional role of being a carer to a vulnerable adult at the end of his or her life.

These personal stories echo the rich variety of examples throughout the book, and they point to finding the space and making the mutual connection to tell our stories, find fresh voices and rethink our narratives. Cognitive Analytic Therapy (Ryle & Kerr, 2020; Hepple & Sutton, 2004; Potter, 2020) is tailor made for such work with its ideas of lifelong emotional roles which we give and take from each other (reciprocal roles) and the snags, traps and dilemmas – already introduced in the preceding chapter by Liz McCormick, and in her book (2017) – and different levels of managing and orchestrating a sense of self.

The emphasis in this chapter is on finding our voices and telling our unique and shared life stories from the vantage point of what it means to be in the later stages of life. However, everything written here applies equally to all stages of adult life. Adults don't stop being adults as they get old. One challenge is not to take to heart the dominant narratives of ageism still current in society, and to find new stories for our changing circumstances of status, health and the growing frailty of our bodies along with the questions of existence, loss and finality as we pass on to the next generations. In later life, we have a chance to retell our stories and recover, rethink and revise or reaffirm the narratives that have shaped our lives individually or collectively and, importantly, we have space for new stories and narratives.

This chapter also keeps in mind that, here at the end of the first quarter of the 21st century, some of the societal narratives that we older people were born with, the middle of the previous century, no longer hold sway. At the point of writing this chapter, now in my mid-70s, it feels clear that both locally and globally the grand narratives of religion, politics, identity, gender, ethnicity, sexuality and class are challenged and exposed. Progress, nostalgia, innovation and reaction are set against each other. Psychologically and socially, we are in a great narrative transition. Olga Tokarczuk, the Polish winner of the Nobel Prize for literature (2019) put her finger on it:

> 'We lack the language, we lack the points of view, the metaphors, the myths and new fables. Yet we do see frequent attempts to harness rusty, anachronistic narratives that cannot fit the future, no doubt on the assumption that an old something is better than a new nothing or trying in this way to deal with the limitations of our own horizons. In a word, we lack new ways of telling the story of the world.'

To borrow Olga Tokarczuk's words, we need new ways of telling the story of ourselves both locally and globally in the world, and this means new narratives. In later life, we need to tell and retell our stories to each other and to the younger generations in search of new understanding, stories that connect us to our common humanity.

The chapter concludes by offering the idea of *story power* as a general benefit of talking with a map alongside problem-solving, stress relief and healing. Story power is the recovery, or discovery for the first time, of narrative curiosity, compassion and competence within ourselves and with each other. It is a mutual power since there is no story without the voices of an author and reader, a speaker and a listener. Story power is the capacity to trust and share the feeling of being more one's own author and more able to find and allow narrative freedom in ourselves and others. It is a power that can sustain us in later life and which we can only give ourselves by giving it and allowing it in others. It is a reflective, narrative, relational and conversational awareness and competence.

Cognitive Analytic Therapy and maps

I use the tools of Cognitive Analytic Therapy (CAT) to make word maps of our conversations. I say it will help me listen. Detailed therapeutic mechanisms of change using mapping have been identified and described (Potter, 2020; 2022).

We learn how and what to feel in our early years with parents, carers and siblings at home, at school, in the playground. As indicated by the toy cowboys and Indians story, we process and work out our learning through conversations with and within ourselves. We learn what amounts to a mental landscape or personal ideology that becomes second nature to us, and different approaches to therapy explore this in terms of core beliefs, schemas, patterns of attachment and identity solutions. In CAT, we have a simplified way of getting to the heart of this complex and often-buried early experience. We identify on paper emotional roles that were central to our primary relationship in early life, and which we took upon ourselves or seeped into us to become how we saw and felt the world, and how those ways of seeing a feeling still remain with us. They are called reciprocal roles in CAT, to highlight how the emotional tone and social agenda of what others do to us, we do to ourselves and to others.

To put it another way, we tend to do the dances within ourselves that our parents, our teachers and our brothers and sisters did with us, and, as we do them, we learn the music and make the steps our own. For better or worse, they are the only dances we know, and we find and maintain a sense of who we are through them. These are the dances of relating described in the preceding chapter. They can be freeing, liberating and validating, or they can be hurtful, restrictive and disorganizing of our sense of self and others. Or they are a confusing mix of both.

When mapping out as we talk, we are trying to reconnect with the early experience of these powerful emotional roles and see how they shaped the narratives we lived by in the present and in the past. We map them out as a call and response, or push and pull, between a top action (or doing end) and a bottom feeling (or done to end) as in the 'Doing and Feeling' layout in Figures 3.1 and 3.2 below. We take care to map from inside the real and remembered experiences of specific stories so as to help the story and its narratives be visible. Mostly, we are made of several connected or contrasting and conflicting emotional roles. Sometimes, the emotional roles are obvious ones to us, like *striving to please demanding and loving parents* and *only feeling loved if achieving and meeting their demands.* But the emotional roles are often buried deep in the past and we begin to know them indirectly from the surface of our behaviour or through our patterns of coping with ourselves and managing others. We can open a journey of exploration with them with the aid of words on paper in the form of a map or diagram. Learning to do this together is the bread and butter of CAT therapy.

In CAT we summarize these everyday coping patterns as the steps within and between the emotional roles we play. We call them traps, dilemmas and snags.

Traps

A *trap* describes a narrow way of thinking that works along the lines of 'I can cope with these feelings or this situation but *only if* I think more narrowly, like this'. For example, if I am feeling hurt because of feelings of neglect, then a trap might be to think that only if I am pleasing and attentive to others will I be OK. The trap leads to a narrow range of responses and, in pleasing others, I may be adding self-neglect to the feeling of neglect from others. A trap is like an attempt to escape a difficult situation that keeps us stuck in it like a self-defeating circle, wherein we end up at the doing end or the feeling end (Figure 3.1), or pinball between both. We hang on to such a pattern because it is the pattern (dance – narrative) we learned, and it is a kind of attachment solution for our identity as the familiar way we know ourselves to be with others. Traps have an addictive and habitual quality, like having a cup of tea in the morning, and it is curious that, when we are reflecting on our own, they don't seem so compelling, but when interacting with others we find ourselves doing them as if on autopilot. This emphasis on the context of how we act as individuals is important. We follow patterns such as traps because they are the narratives that others expect to know us by and recruit us into.

Figure 3.1: Mapping a trap

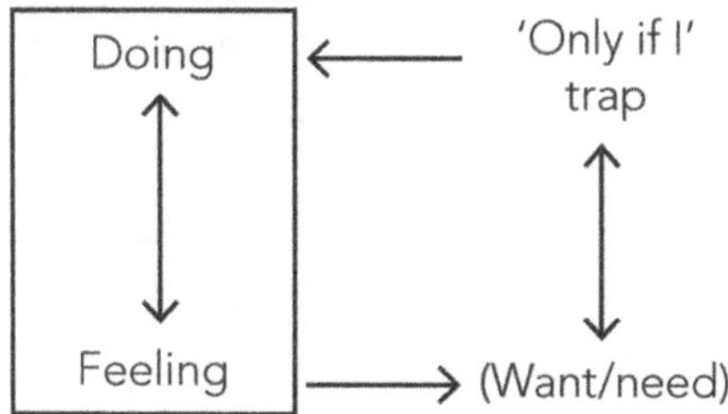

So, traps are maintained because they partly work to give us an emotional identity – for example, in the pleasing others trap, I see myself as a nice person. In mapping out one or more traps about our ways of giving meaning to how we relate and respond, the aim is not to blame or shame ourselves or try to get rid of the trap, but to be compassionate towards the history behind it and the context around it, and to find shifts in changing its weight or intensity or finding alternatives to it, and ways of out of it before it kicks in. The emphasis in CAT is not just on the thinking part but on the interactive whole of the pattern. It is not so much saying 'change your thinking', but that we should try to see the whole dance and change your relationship with the dance, and the thinking will change. A trap is a simplified narrative of relating that we can hold in mind across several stories and situations. It helps to write the trap out in a single sentence from the map. It can tease out how we live our lives in different places and times.

Dilemmas

A *dilemma* is a pinball behavioural choice of Either-Or: either this behaviour or that behaviour. If I am feeling hurt either I speak up and cause trouble or I stay quiet, keep out of trouble but remain hurt. Both behaviours seem to come back to restrict me and hit me emotionally. Or I pinball between two behaviours coloured by gender, class, culture and ethnicity or accent – *as a girl, either I speak up and get silenced as loud and shouty or I stay quiet and am seen as sweet but have no voice of my own*. Or, *as a boy, I act tough and get excused and indulged as just like a boy or I show tenderness and am seen as soft and judged as a cissy.* In these examples, as in Figure 3.2, there is no middle way, and the therapeutic and reflective conversation is a chance to discover middle ways and be open to the social forces behind the split and divided behaviour.

Figure 3.2: Either-Or dilemma

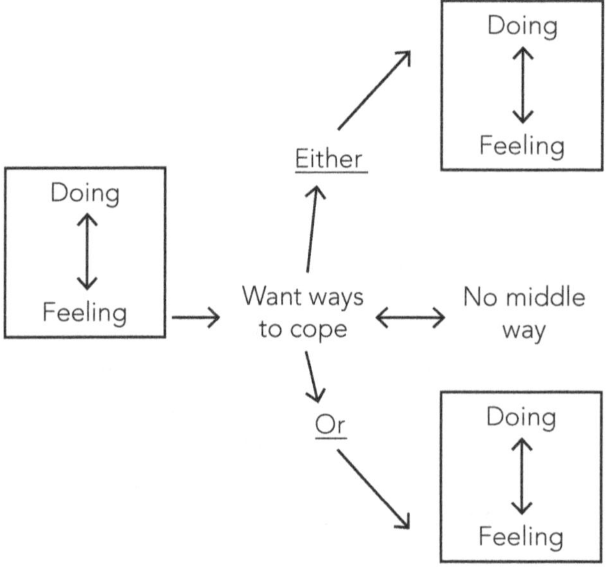

Dilemmas can define our group membership and our inner world in binary ways and give rise to attitudes of prejudice and racism, as in, either we are in *this group* and behave like this, in ways that are superior, or you are in *that group* and behave in ways that we judge as inferior and other than us. One option may dominate my way of relating because early on in life I learned by the rules of gender or class or ethnicity or disability to never opt for one of the behaviours. For example, always being polite because it was not safe to get noisy or angry. The forbidden or buried side of the dilemma can be a ghost role or behaviour, and we know the steps to its dance but have long denied that it is part of who we are. A dilemma in later life might be either I am pleasant and cheerful and easy to look after but then, as a result, I am dull – and ignored as boring, or I am interesting but stubborn and disagreeable and a pain to care for'. When we wish to assert ourselves, the idea of being stubborn and disagreeable in the eyes of others may haunt us and ghost us into keeping quiet. These ghost roles are easier to rework and understand by mapping them out.

To summarize, dilemmas are habitual lines of behaviour or action and are usefully mapped out as patterns that we carry within us as fixed narratives from the past but that are also narratives in our culture and in the organization of society. If we can map these out with compassion and curiosity together – especially if we are in helping and caring roles or as neighbours – we can find alternative behaviours in the middle group between and outside the pinball effect of either doing this or doing that.

Snags

Finally, in CAT, there is the idea of the *snag* as a pattern of relating to self and society that is driven by a *Yes-But* response as in. Yes, I am doing OK and getting my needs met, but something or someone will pop up to disallow or block me. For example, I am making progress in getting the care and treatment I need, *yes*. But you are jumping the queue, the others will say, or you are neglecting the grandchildren. Or, yes I am offering to help with the family and the grandchildren *But*, the other will say, we don't want you to overdo it. *Yes-But* is like a block or glass ceiling that comes from within us or from outside through society's prejudices or values and stops something helpful or worthwhile in its tracks. These can be lifelong narratives that haunt us: Yes, but girls or boys don't do that. Yes, but you were not very good at drawing at primary school so don't try that painting class. Yes, it would be lovely to visit cousins and reminisce, but old people don't gad about or make a fuss.

When we map and talk, our words on paper and our diagrams are messy, regardless of how many times we have done it. We scribble and scrawl our words to keep up with and in tune with the conversation. However, the templates are useful to have in mind as neat versions that might guide us and help us tidy up a messy map and make new connections.

Figure 3.3: 'Yes But' Snag

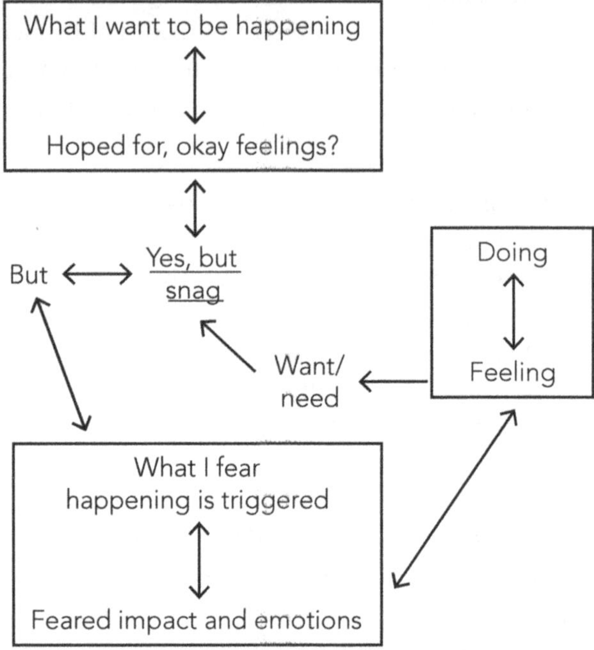

First example: Jane's 'triple whammy' story linking a trap, a dilemma and a snag

Here is Jane's example, where the shift between coping in the form of a trap, dilemma or snag is highlighted. Jane was talking about feeling neglected by her children and by the staff in the care home and by the hospital for not confirming her appointment (summed up as the emotional role at point 1 on the map Figure 3.4). She felt hurt and neglected, feelings which had powerful echoes from her childhood, but her main narrative then, as now, was to get care by meeting other people's needs (point 2 on the map) which, as we mapped it out as a pattern, showed that, in the process, there was a trap in which she would also neglect herself alongside the neglect from others. It was voiced like this between us: 'What others do to me, I then do to myself'. But not all the time, because Jane was also pulled and pushed around by a *dilemma* of either being self-reliant and feeling strong while looking after others but alone and lonely (point 7 on the map), or being needily demanding (now in ill-health) of the responses of others (point 8 on the map), which tended to leave her feeling partly cared for but dependent, vulnerable and exposed. As we mapped out these patterns of relating within herself and with the world, we were looking for ways of being outside them, softening them or having alternatives to them. Just talking in this way stopped her blaming herself and gave her some compassion and curiosity. We identified a third and deeper pattern that came from within her that we called her 'Yes-But snag' (point 3 on the map in Figure 3.4). Jane said she had learned it from her mum and dad, and generations of deference to those above them. It worked as on the map in Figure 3.4. When Jane made moves to be noticed, she did get appreciated and responded to, but something deep within her jumped out and scolded or shamed her, as if forbidding her and people like her to speak up and ask for attention. Sometimes, awareness of snags like this can help weaken their hold and lead to a better understanding of their place in the society we have grown up in and lived our lives in.

Figure 3.4: Linking a trap, dilemma and snag for Jane

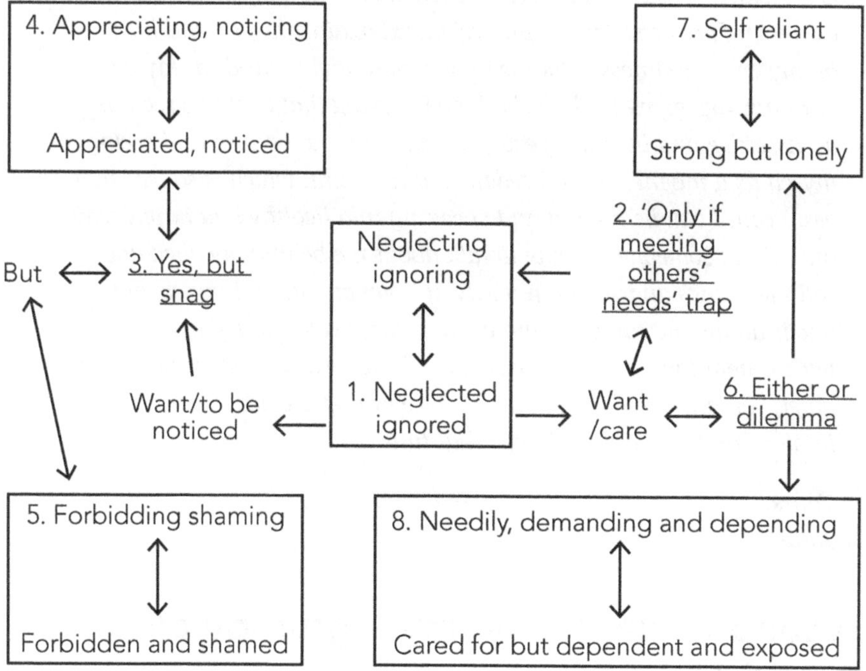

Bits of therapeutic writing to parts of the map

As we talk and map and recap, we are looking for break-out and break-through moments when or where something different happens. These are the moments that point to narrative freedom and change the story in the future. One big opportunity in this direction, there and then in the therapy or discussion, is to write to all or part of the map. Writing, even a sentence or two, to capture one pattern on the map can help connect with it in more helpful, reflective and emotionally focused ways. Jane wrote the following right there in the session in front of the map. When she read it out and we revised and re-read it, she felt more power over her story.

> ***Dear Triple Whammy Map*** *(especially the yes-but bit) I do feel neglected and ignored but I can cope with it if I understand my part in it. Like the map says, I am wired to meet other people's needs, and I don't see that as a trap with others but can see how I trap myself in it if it is the only dance that I allow myself. The trouble is, if I get stuck in the strong, heroic, self-reliant me, up there in the Either-Or dilemma, then I get so cross and frustrated that I can be demanding and then fear shifting into an exposed and vulnerable moaning, 'she is a moaner' position. I need to see whether there are other ways of expressing my needs or if I am prejudiced against myself and hard on my own neediness. What is wrong with having needs at my age, or at any age going back to childhood? Saying that could be seen as an assertive and liberating exit from expecting to be seen and seeing myself as a moaner. Then I see the crunch point, which is so true that yes, I can. I can be noticed and speak up in a healthy and happy way, but I think someone is going to talk about me behind my back and call me names and say I am needy. If I pay attention, I notice that no one is doing that, and it is more like a ghost voice or a ghost role going back generations. Having needs is needy, asserting needs is bad. Keep quiet, you are forbidden to have a voice and give voice to your basic human needs. I want to change that tune.*
>
> ***Yours,***
> ***Jane***

Second example: Jimmy – grumpy old so-and-so

Jimmy comes into my therapy room, sits down and looks at me as if to size me up and then looks away out the window and says, 'I am grumpy old so-and-so'. He talks for a while in this vein. I think to myself, we men tend to do this. We give the headline and plant the narrative upfront before we tell any stories. Are we afraid of the spontaneous power of stories and memories to disrupt our preferred adult narratives? We tell set jokes and we banter. Now, as our session gets underway, my thought is that Jimmy is protecting himself or me by controlling our conversation by telling me the narrative to listen for and making sure, for both of us, that there is zero storytelling spontaneity. So I dither, pen in hand – usefully and constructively, I hope – because I don't want to fall into my own *psychotherapist knows best* narrative. After a while, Jimmy looks at me, dithering, and says, 'Are you all right mate?' It is as if he fears I have no narrative to offer at all. I say, 'Yes, I am sorry, I was just hesitating over my thoughts. We don't have to rush, do we?' I feel a bit grumpy, too.

I ask for his permission (I say it will help me listen) to write down his opening statement in the middle of a blank sheet of paper in front of us – 'Me a grumpy old so-and-so' – and circle it, and put a question mark beside it. I think his self-description as grumpy is a lifelong response to something painful or a mix of feelings which later we fill out as the *emotional impact* at the bottom end of the grey box (agitated, useless, needy and sad) and then find some sense of what has been going on (done by him and or done by others) at the *action* end at the top of the grey box on the left. He prods the question mark. 'What's that for?' with a bit of a grumpy tone to his voice. 'Not to jump to conclusions.' I say that I want to talk and hear some of the stories from his life first before I simply agree with him that he is a grumpy so-and-so. I say that, if I react to that (pointing to the phrase 'grumpy'), it would be like just reading the newspaper headlines and not the stories underneath. He smiles and says, 'But that is exactly what I do with the newspapers'. I want him and I to get inside the idea of being grumpy and bring it alive in terms of how it traps him, snags his relationships and narrows his behaviour into an Either-Or dilemma of doing X or doing Y to no satisfactory end.

'Me too', I say, and add that we do live by headlines and banter and quick thinking, and we gain by it, but it also costs us. We think it is smart, but actually it can make our relationships shallow and limit our understanding. It closes our stories down before we have opened them up. He sort of agrees and we chat on like this about how men tell stories. I think I am trying to create a storytelling space and a storytelling relationship that is open and not already narrated. The words in Figure 3.5 on paper bring us alongside each other and break the ice. Our tone of voice is varied and not grumpy. The words on paper are like little way markers around which the conversation is circulating and growing.

Figure 3.5: The grumpy trap

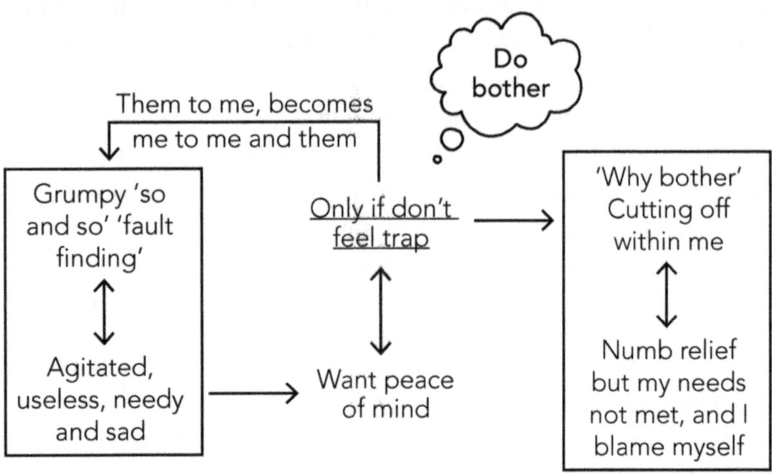

After a while, I suggest an idea about storytelling. I suggested that Jimmy tells me a story that shows him as a grumpy old so-and-so in his view. And then tell me one that you are not sure what it shows or where it goes. He tells me of not wanting to see his grandchildren and being cross with his wife for going to see them. We agree that was a grumpy story but get something else from it. There is a sad and needy and agitated state (the bottom end of the grey box in Figure 3.5) which the *grumpy so-and-so* pattern keeps at bay. Once we touch this, he tells me of not being able to sit down on the floor with the children, and even worse, not being able to get up and keep up with them because of his arthritis. His tone of voice is sad, but not grumpy. The second story is about playing dominoes with his grandchildren and their joy at finding a game just in the zone of what they can do. It is evidently his joy, too, because not only can he do it and enjoy it, but it takes him back a lifetime of playing with his siblings and his grandma 70 years before. I say, perhaps what we are doing now in our conversation is a bit like playing dominoes?

With mapping to help us, the patterns on paper don't just point upwards to an overarching narrative, but sideways to other stories from other times in life. On paper, we were opening up space for reflection and curiosity between the grumpy state of self and the stories within it. We soon agreed that his key response felt in the moment and carried with him at times from childhood was *why bother?* It was a painful and emotional phrase. I wanted to say, just impulsively from my heart, but you do bother. You are here, you have lived a full life. But I didn't need to because he pointed to the words why bother and, looking at me, said, 'I *do bother*'. I put *I do bother* at the top of the sheet of paper as the hopeful and good place to come back to and not lose sight of. We talked on and off the map for a while. Jimmy described patterns of *If not grumpy then alive, but getting into fights and messing about with people and jobs and letting people down*. They fit his grumpy narrative but there is something else they are hiding. There is a second narrative or theme. He is critical of himself for being like that. We are developing narrative awareness and narrative freedom. In the next few sessions, we write to *Dear Grumpy So-and-So* and write out the pattern with which we have started. He can see it as a narrative that comes into so many of his life stories but now it has new and different angles and lines to it which he is more confident talking about.

> ***Dear Grumpy, needy and fault finding.*** *You are what I am often like, and I can tell you I learned it from my dad. He was like that to us kids and to my mum. It made us feel obligated and needed but useless and always on edge like it says at the heart of the map. I have been in this relationship with myself for so many years and, just like my dad, I have dragged people into it. People that I love or loved. I cut myself off as a child and do it now to cope and I feel numb inside and can appear like that to others. The map says it plain and simple. I can't help it, even though deep down I want to help myself out of it or let others in. I am either in a grumpy state and accusing myself and feel useless and guilty, or in a 'why bother' state and am safe but cut off. It feels a relief to have some clues about the run around that this does to me. I feel kinder to myself and maybe I can get out of it. What really mattered was that moment of saying I do bother, and I guess I was bothering in the sessions. He was bothering as well. I needed that.*
>
> ***Yours,***
> ***Jimmy (not so grumpy)***

The mapping and the talking gave enough of a necessarily simplified framework for Jimmy to have more elaborate and complex conversations with himself and talk with others about alternative lines of thinking and have interest in other people's patterns.

Third example: Mary's dream that keeps her real

Mary was near the end of her life, but something kept her in touch with vitality and gave her a handle on reality. She enjoyed a lifelong capacity for dreams. Her mother saw it as a childhood indulgence – 'Your head's in the clouds, you need your feet on the ground, dreams won't get you through life'. But they did, and in her final years they still do. Daydreams that got her to sleep at night and sometimes took on the quality of dreams from deep sleep. Mary would talk of the dreams as if they were an important and real part of her, but if firmly challenged by someone in authority, she would say in a cross and hurt way that of course she knew they were her 'wistfulness', and why not? Everyone who cared for her went along with her dream world or woe betide them. Mary's only daughter and grown-up grandchildren, and her two great-grandchildren, were in Australia, and in healthy times during her later life she had made two visits, much to her and their delight. Now, in reality, another visit was never on the cards, but Mary daily told those who saw her or cared for her that she would soon be booking her ticket, or that the ticket was booked, and bags would need to be packed.

Conversations went on at length as to what would need taking, presents to buy, how she would survive the arduous journey and the joys and perils of the long flight down under. It was a half pretence that helped nourish lots of side stories, memories and an outstanding narrative of looking forward. It did important psychological and spiritual work. There was a deep attachment narrative about loving her children and grandchildren tinged with joy and sadness and going on a journey, as well as a more immediate narrative about having some immediate business for discussion. Not only did it cheer Mary up, but it also gave her a focus and lots of starter conversations that could then link to reminiscing and to detailed descriptions of her grandchildren and her daughter *who was no longer a spring chicken herself, truth be told, and who, according to Mary, is too old to travel back to England.* A detached observer might say Mary should not be encouraged in her dream, but mapping out this central conversation in her final days showed a deeper truth. We need our dreams to have a second or third narrative outside of immediate reality. They need gentle reality testing, but they don't need puncturing. Someone inadvertently saw her passport in her drawer and said it was a lovely picture but was now out of date. Mary was suddenly crestfallen but responded with scorn – don't be ridiculous put it away. Denial can be a protective factor.

Figure 3.6: Mary's dream

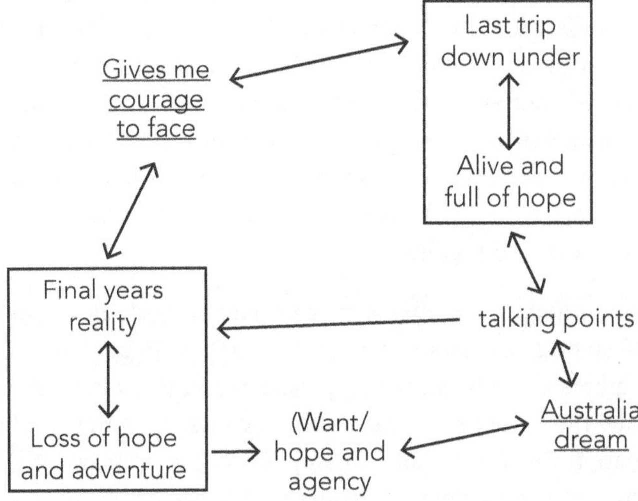

For some the idea of a protective factor is judged as a denial of reality if it is based on investing hope in something that can't happen such as a trip to Australia or is untestable such as the afterlife. But if we can dwell therapeutically in the spaces between what's really real and what is dreamed up to be real then we may gain narrative freedom. Above all, it may give texture to our conversation and help us see there is more than one story at the end of life, as highlighted by the pattern here, as in Figure 3.6 above. When life takes on the form in which all our stories seem to be imprisoned in one final narrative, then we need a second or a third narrative to step out and be in between narratives. It is better to have a second narrative that is dreamlike than no narrative at all. We can't do this on our own and need others to help us. It is easier with a map.

Fourth example: Bihar's empathy trap

Bihar was an assistant manager in a care home who had come back to her old job after a time raising her children. She had worked there when younger and had enjoyed it. She was generous with her time and open to the residents. She could divide her working days into good days and bad days. Good days were when everyone seemed to get out on the right side of the bed. There was cooperation and a feeling that residents and staff were working together. On bad days, though, someone could kick someone else off emotionally and, like a contagion, everyone ended up feeling on edge and not knowing why, and look for something or someone to blame, or blaming themselves until it was too much, and something had to give. There was a rule, with which Bihar didn't entirely agree, not to get too involved. The rule was not to join the dance and not to let the residents see the white of your eyes (i.e., the fear or vulnerability). For Bihar, there was a line along which she walked back and forth every day – at one end was far too much empathy, and at the other end was too little. We called it the empathy trap, if you let yourself feel too much for someone and their emotional distress or difficulties.

The empathy trap goes like this: someone 'has to care', and if no one cares, I will step up and do the caring. I know how to do it, so I will take it all on and others stand back, which pushes me to be even more involved and I become the heroic carer trapped by my own empathy and by others leaving me to it. Bihar saw that a dilemma was also in play – one of either being caring and risking being over-involved, or being cheery and distant but too detached, emotionally. Empathy is a delicate two-way feeling for self and for others and, in an organization providing services and care, it is a juggling act of turn-taking, involvement and detachment. The reflective capacity to sustain such awareness is more easily nurtured through team discussions with mapping to help draw out shared patterns.

Top tips for mapping as we talk

- Have a big sheet of paper or an A4 notebook open to double the size and space of the sheet.
- Say it will help us listen if we track on paper the keywords for the feelings, ideas and relationships that come up so we can remember and go over them together when we recap where the conversation has got to.
- Every so often, to highlight the shared and open process of listening, stop the conversation and recap with the words spread out on paper to see the links and gaps in patterns of relating and feeling from the stories and narratives being shared.
- Also recap with the word map to construct softer or sharper versions or exits from fixed narratives and develop new ways of retelling old stories.
- Use the words on the paper as markers to talk about how the conversation is going – what helps and hinders – and to explore ways to change tack and keep going when the conversation feels fragile or confronting.

- When the conversations with the mapping process are more established, each of you should write a five-minute letter to one part of the map that troubles or inspires you.
- Read them out to each other and respect and recognize how bits of writing from the map or deliberate stopping and recapping with the map are also a moment to hear your voices as the gateways to hidden feelings, meanings and connections.
- Mapping, writing and voicing are all multi-sensory, multi-media experiences that activate different parts of the brain in different orchestrations. Don't rush, but give yourself time to be in and among the mix of this palette of experiences. An important process of memory reconsolidation is taking place.
- Remember that the map is just words on paper and not some special document carrying the truth – it is only as good as the conversation it enables.
- Use the map as an analogical or mirror space alongside the conversation, which is to say use it as whatever you want to call it: a climbing frame, a safety net, a navigation aid and an extended shared working memory space.
- Don't map a person, or a world view, but map your way around one story of a moment and the people and the world and the thinking and the ideologies will come into view.

Story power: A prescription for later life

The preceding examples show the small steps to building the power to hold a story open long enough to develop relational awareness and reflective capacity and narrative freedom. It is the ability to hover and shimmer between different life stories and soften the old and troublesome narratives enough to step out of them and claim a narrative freedom and vitality in the present. That way, our shared storytelling has a chance to sparkle with honesty and authenticity and we can give room for the relational mental health we need to survive as a species on a habitable planet.

Clients like the ones described fictionally in this chapter often say something like, 'In the end, you have not made me totally better, but you have given me the power to tell my own stories, to hold in mind different points of view, and not be stuck in one voice or narrative'. I wonder with them whether this story power was something we had the best taste of in late childhood, if we were lucky, but then had crammed out of us in secondary school and teenage subcultures. I regard it as a process of becoming our own authors with narrative freedom to enter into our own and other people's stories. What are the ingredients that help enable this through mapping and talking? Well, that is a big question, but for this chapter they can be summarized as the following:

- **Getting involved or standing back.** When we tell our life stories, we are inviting each other in, to participate and empathize and travel alongside us. Mapping as we talk allows us to move in more closely or hold back and see things from a distance. If we do this for each other, it is easier to live it within ourselves and feel for or stand back from different sides of ourselves and the different qualities of narrative they allow or limit. We are all made up of several parts, roles, identities, stories and narratives, and however we define them, a key quality is to do what Philip Bromberg aptly called standing in the spaces (Bromberg, 1998). When we get involved, we get entangled and dance to the tunes of each other's narratives often without realizing it or knowing how to discuss it. One of our earliest developmental skills as infants and toddlers is that of taking turns, and in taking turns, we allow involvement and standing back.
- **Shimmering-feeling.** When we talk, there is the opportunity to go with the push and pull of mixed feelings and ambivalence about the direction and intensity of emotion. We need to help each other notice, name and negotiate when to cool things down, hot things up or separate out emotions and feelings that have become welded onto each other through the heat or pace of their expression. Our storytelling power depends on a shared feeling for emotions of hurt and anger, pride or delight and superiority, guilt and shame, desire and control expressed in words and gestures or carried in our bodies in their different contexts.
- **Hovering-thinking.** There is a quality of thought that might best be called relational thinking because it can hold in mind movement between picture-detail, past-present, my ideas and your ideas, surface and depth, true and false, and thereby work together in making links, tolerating gaps not going binary between now and then, here and there, self and others. Hovering is a kind of constructive dithering in search

of new meanings or new angles on old narratives so something new or important or old and intrusive can be enquiringly and compassionately brought to awareness, relived and reworked.

- **Authoring-owning.** There is a necessary fragility, sensitivity and delicacy to our personal conversations when they are open. When we stop talking at each other or as we navigate our hopes and fears, we fear loss of meaning, exposure or shame or perhaps more deeply still a loss of authorship when I don't know what I am saying. The gift of a good conversation is to feel an ownership and a growing authorship both separately and together. When we are finding and owning our words and we are taking possession of the conversation, we are ultimately taking possession of ourselves. Authorship is felt as having authority. A story freely told but carefully listened to with feelings and ideas noticed, named and negotiated is an experience of good authority and narrative coherence.

Summary

This chapter has shown the specific craft of mapping out on paper the words that show our patterns of relating and give narrative meaning to our life stories as we tell them and reflect upon the telling of them. It has placed these skills as the mediator between story and narrative. Hopefully, the examples have spoken for themselves. The chapter ends with a plea and a claim. The plea is for a society that gives more attention to building our story power (what is word power for if not for that?) or narrative competence and freedom. The claim is that mapping and writing interactively as guided by CAT tools can help build our reflective capacity and relational awareness and thereby give elbow to our story power. Our later years in life, not unlike our later years of childhood, may be a second experience of increasing or recovering our story power. So, I propose *story power* as the freedom and right to tell and retell our life stories in a wholehearted and shared search for understanding and the shared sense of authorship it can bring in later life. We are going to need it during the great transitions locally and globally that are now around us. Like elders from time immemorial, we have something to contribute in this way by looking back and looking forward at the same time.

Chapter 4: Finding a compassionate life story

Alistair Gaskell

'Life can only be understood backwards, but it must be lived forwards.'

(Soren Kirkegaard)

In this chapter, I would like to explore the judgements that we make and hold onto about ourselves, in particular the ideas that we often have, that we are 'failures' or 'losers', or a 'burden' to those around us, or that we are 'useless' or 'weak' or 'unlovable'. For some, these are fleeting ideas surrounded by more appreciative or caring ones. But for rather many people, in all stages of life, they can be ideas that stick with us, that we cannot avoid or forget, that form the backdrop for the whole of our lives. Sadly, at times, they are an important part of why a person might choose to end their life.

These ideas are by no means unique to later life, we can and do hold them at any age, but perhaps they can have a particular force and poignancy as we get older. If we see ourselves as a 'failure' in the earlier part of our life, we may hold on to the thought that perhaps things will change, but later on we may rightly or wrongly feel that the course of our life has been set and cannot be changed. To have an idea that our life is not failing but has failed is a particular kind of torment.

Within the dominant Cognitive Behavioural Therapy (CBT) model, our relationship with ourselves is conceptualized mainly in terms of our thoughts or beliefs. The founder of modern CBT, Aaron Beck (Beck *et al*, 1979), described negative beliefs about oneself as part of the 'cognitive triad' of negative beliefs (along with negative beliefs about the world and the future), which he considered to be at the heart of depression. More generally, such beliefs are seen as being part of low self-esteem, which can often be a lifelong problem and a vulnerability factor for many mental health problems (Fennel, 1999).

Sometimes cognitive behavioural therapists will consider the root of such beliefs, but often it is not thought necessary to trace the beliefs back within our life story and wider social context. Instead, we may be encouraged to identify and label our thoughts, to challenge them, and think about ways to replace them with alternative beliefs.

Self-compassion

A separate but related approach comes from Paul Gilbert and his colleagues, who married cognitive behavioural ideas with Buddhist traditions to create an approach Gilbert termed Compassion-Focused Therapy. He quotes the social psychologist Mark Leary who wrote a book entitled *The Curse of the Self*. Gilbert argues that our ability to think about our 'self' comes from the evolution of a 'new' part of the brain able to observe and reflect on our mental activity. The 'curse of the self' is that this ability opens us up to comparisons and evaluations that cause distress to the 'old' emotional part of the brain.

Gilbert argues that we need to gain a different, more compassionate perspective on this type of painful self-evaluation. When we tell ourselves we are 'stupid' because, for instance, of something we said, we fail to realize how insignificant what we said was. He draws on Buddhist traditions that tell us that the self is largely an illusion and suggests that it is helpful to step back from our judgements of ourselves and think about them in a different context.

He writes about the way that our minds are formed in the context of 'accidents of genetics and history' and the powerful influence of the context in which we happen to be born and a few years later 'find ourselves'. Each of us is 'a little wavelet on a vast sea that rises and falls'. Viewed in this context, 'it makes little sense to blame ourselves for some of our feelings, motives, desires or abilities, or lack of them, or for how things turned out' (Gilbert, 2009).

I think there is a profound truth in this. It can be incredibly helpful to understand our insignificance within the vastness of the world, let alone the universe. One of my clients recently said to me, after decades of struggling with the belief that he did not deserve to have been born, that he had come to realize that this belief was not just wrong but that it was nonsensical. It made no more sense than the idea that a rabbit did not deserve to have been born and he could see how irrelevant the concept of deserving to be born was to a rabbit's life.

Gilbert goes on to offer us exercises, based partly on Buddhist traditions of mindfulness and meditation and partly on using the parts of our emotional brain, that he calls the soothing and contentment system, to practice creating a more compassionate relationship with ourselves (Gilbert *et al*, 2010). A related approach is described by Liz McCormick in Chapter 2 of this book, and such exercises can be extremely helpful in allowing us to reach a state of mind where we are able to accept ourselves and find more compassionate thoughts and feelings.

But while these approaches are very useful, and may be the right approaches for many people, they often leave unexamined the question of where ideas such as 'I am useless' or 'I am a failure' might come from and why they often seem so hard to dislodge. As described in Chapter 1, later life is often a time of life review, when we want to make sense of our life and our place in the world and who we are as a person. This is very much in line with my experience as a clinical psychologist working with older people. There is very often a desire to understand why we feel the way we do.

So, I would like to pose a question: if we would like to reach a point of acceptance and self-compassion, what is it helpful for us to understand? My attempt at an answer will focus on two things. First, I would like to consider cultural ideas about such things as success and failure, and why they are such important and powerful ideas. Second, I would like to think about how we understand the adversities that we have experienced in our lives; particularly how we often fail to understand the influence that adversity has had on the way that our lives have unfolded, and so unfairly apply to ourselves our culture's ideas of failure. To do this, I would like to explore the idea of 'voices'.

Voices

> *'The older you get, the more voices you get in the back of your head.'*
>
> (Robert Jackson Bennett, *American Elsewhere*)

For CAT therapists, one way of thinking about ideas such as 'I am a failure' or 'I am useless', is that they are utterances from an internal voice, a voice with which we are talking to ourselves.

When thinking about this kind of voice, we are not quite using the word literally. They may not be something that we literally say in our minds or that we hear. The most important thing about this kind of voice is that it is a message that we send to ourselves. For some people they may indeed be spoken and heard, but for others they have a different quality. For one of my clients, the 'voice' was visual. She spoke about picturing a neon sign above her head with the word 'Failure' lit up for all to see.

These voices do not occur in isolation. As described in Chapter 2, CAT theory suggests that our relationship with ourselves is connected with the patterns we have experienced in relationships with others, particularly in our early life. One way of describing this is through the idea of reciprocal roles. Another, broadly similar, way of putting this is that our voice to ourselves is connected to voices that were used towards us in the past and that are also used in the present. Again, in this context, a 'voice' can be both literal things that people have said and more subtle messages about who we are as a person and what our place is in the world. In CAT theory, it is thought that we 'internalize' voices that have been used towards us in our relationships with others .

As with other kinds of psychotherapy, CAT therapists have often been interested in the voices and messages coming from our parents when we were young, but the same process can take place at other times in our lives. If we have a partner or an important friend who is often critical of us, we may internalize this. Additionally, voices do not need to come from specific people – we can internalize the voice of a group of people, or a voice coming more generally from the culture around us. Again, an alternative way to describe this would be as a reciprocal role between ourselves and the culture surrounding us.

Cultural voices

I think these cultural voices are easy to underestimate. The culture that we live in is something shared, and while it changes continually, the slow pace of change is not easy to notice. Unless we experience a move from one culture to another, we may not notice the messages that our culture gives us that 'go without saying' about what it is to be a good or successful or loveable person. When we express something like 'I am a failure', we are speaking not only to ourselves but to 'the wider world' – that is, the culture that we inhabit. Expressing it, we are taking for granted that it is possible to divide people along the lines of 'failures' or 'successes', and that it is important which category we fit into. I think it also takes for granted that these things are *morally* important. That is, that being 'a success' somehow makes us a good person and 'a failure' a bad person. These ideas are not natural, they are the product of cultural values.

We inhabit a culture, in Britain and I think most of the Western world, in which evaluation is all around us. We are surrounded by signals of our status, in where we live, what job we have, the car we drive, the clothes that we wear, and the relationships we have or perhaps don't have with others. We are usually in very little doubt about our place within this culture, whether we are high or low status, how secure that status is, and whether it is rising or falling. It has probably always been a little bit like that. Most human cultures (and some animal cultures) seem to have some element of ranking and comparison. But when comparing cultures, modern Western culture, as well as being very competitive and status-conscious, is often characterized as more individualistic. There seems to be more emphasis on our identity as individuals rather than as members of a group, by comparison with both more traditional cultures of our past and modern-day cultures of East Asian countries (Hofstede *et al*, 2010).

Of course, our identity is not solely determined by where we stand in the social 'pecking order'. There are other aims in life which are somewhat (although rarely completely) removed from the pursuit of material success. We can pursue a career or try to build a happy family life. We can gain satisfaction from helping others or fighting for a cause. Yet these are all enterprises where our cultural fascination with success and failure is hard to avoid completely, and if things go wrong, for instance if we have a 'failed' marriage or a poor relationship with our children, our culture's voice tends to tell us that this is our failure.

As I write this chapter, one of the main news stories in the UK is the very tragic death, apparently by suicide, of Ruth Perry, a primary school headteacher. Her death came in the context of an inspection of her school by Ofsted, whose role is to inspect and grade schools. Her school was due to be downgraded from 'outstanding' to 'inadequate'. In a TV interview, her sister, Julia Waters, said, 'This one word judgement was just destroying thirty-two years of her vocation' (Jeffreys *et al*, 2023). It is not possible and would be wrong to make a judgement about the possibly complex causes of her death, but it illustrates how our culture can consider it normal to make an evaluation that may have a major impact on a person's identity.

One particularly pernicious aspect of our cultural ideas of success and failure is that there seems to be a voice that tells us that, if we succeed, we should take credit for it, and if we fail we can be blamed. Anyone who researches inequality in society will tell you that the advantages and disadvantages that we are born with determine to a great extent where we end up in life in terms of education, work and material wealth (e.g. Braveman *et al*, 2011). Add a dollop of good or bad luck along the way, and very little of it is our doing. But as a culture, we do not seem to want to know this. There seems to be a cultural voice that tells us, 'You get what you deserve'. We hear different forms of it all the time. We may hear about a 'self-made millionaire', or a celebrity who 'chased their dreams' to become a successful singer or footballer, and who perhaps tells us that to succeed you need to 'want it enough'. If we internalize the voice that says we get what we deserve, we don't need to look far for someone to blame when things go wrong.

Finding a fairer narrative about our lives

As is described in Chapter 1, older people, overall, tend to be more contented, better at regulating their emotions and more accepting than younger people. I think this greater acceptance is probably also true of accepting our limitations, and the mistakes and imperfections that make up much of our life stories. However, this greater self-acceptance is by no means universal. In my work as a clinical psychologist with older people, I hear so many stories of self-blame for the way that life has turned out. To the listener, these stories seem to range from slightly to completely unfair. We tell ourselves that we are to blame for things going wrong and fail to notice or to give ourselves any credit for the things that have gone right. It is not enough for someone just to point this out; the self-blaming voice is likely to have been formed and strengthened over many years. But if we put time into reconsidering our life, it can lead to a different story and help us to develop a different voice, and how we speak to ourselves. In CAT, we call this Reformulation. Key to this, is understanding the adversity we have experienced.

Understanding adversity

Life is, in general, pretty challenging, and many of us have experienced adversity which makes these challenges much harder. Yet it is often difficult to think clearly about childhood adversity. The 'you get what you deserve' cultural voice has something to do with this, but on top of this, I think there are cultural voices that are dismissive of our emotional experiences. For those of us growing up in Britain, particularly between about the 1930s to the 1960s, there is a strong cultural voice that tells us we shouldn't dwell on our experiences of adversity and suffering. We shouldn't 'make a fuss'.

Acknowledging suffering is 'feeling sorry for yourself' or 'self-indulgent'. We should just 'get on with it'. Unfortunately, this voice is a hindrance to any attempt to find a fairer perspective on our lives.

In thinking about adversity and its effects on us, it is a fair perspective that we seek. It is not about dramatizing or seeking to paint our experience as unique or special. It is also not about blaming our parents (or anyone else!). There may be times when we have feelings of blame, but those of us who have become parents ourselves will know that it is not necessary to be a bad parent for our children to experience adversity. Adversity can happen at any stage in our lives, but that experienced in childhood may have a particularly profound impact as it happens at a formative stage and when we have the fewest resources to survive it. Childhood adversity has a strong link to many mental and physical health problems and other negative outcomes. It is also remarkably common. One large American study suggested nearly two-thirds of people have experienced adverse childhood events or family dysfunction (Felitti *et al*, 1998).[9] The definition used in this study was fairly narrow, excluding experiences like being bullied, so the true figure is likely to be larger than this.

There are many forms of childhood adversity. We can think about physical, sexual and emotional abuse, such as repeated mockery or criticism. There are also the effects of lack of care, material or emotional, which we sometimes term 'neglect'. We can think of illness, divorce and separation from parents, loss of parents or siblings, mental illness in the family, neurodiversity, which was almost always undiagnosed (and for most older adults today, remains undiagnosed), racial discrimination, forced migration or frequent moves of home. This is quite a list, but even so, it is not exhaustive; there are so many things that can make a childhood harder. The danger of writing this kind of list, though, is that it may encourage our internalized voice that dismisses emotional experience. We may say to ourselves, 'I haven't been through most of those things', or may compare ourselves to children in war zones or in areas going through natural disasters and say, 'I haven't anything to complain about'. If this has gone through your mind, I would encourage acknowledging these voices, but then gently trying to ignore them. What is important is thinking about what we have experienced rather than trying to measure how bad it was. Even relatively small amounts of adversity can have quite profound and long-lasting effects if it interferes with the normal process of emotional development.

Adversity and emotional development

When young children are emotionally well cared for, the natural response to a negative experience is to cry and seek help from an adult, who may help with the cause of the distress but also help us to soothe ourselves. If we are lucky enough to experience such caring, we can internalize a calming, soothing voice, which helps us to deal with distressing situations in our own lives and others'. It helps us to provide the soothing voice needed if we become a parent or carer.

Many types of adversity interfere with this process. There may not be anyone able to hear our distress. We may then internalize a voice saying something like 'no one is interested' or 'you're not important'. That voice will make it hard for us to be interested in our distress later in life or the distress of those that we are caring for. Or the distress may be responded to in a critical, mocking or punitive way, which will lead us to internalize this type of voice and use it on ourselves or others. Sometimes, our distress elicits care, but conditionally; only if the distress is expressed in the 'right' way. For example, we may learn to amplify our distress in order to make it noticeable or minimize it so that it does not overwhelm or elicit a negative response. Sometimes, the response to our distress can be unpredictable, which leads to a great deal of anxiety and confusion about how to respond to distressing situations.

Conditional responses can be some of the most difficult for our emotional development. We may feel that we have to give the response that others want, that we have to be perfect or selfless and undemanding in order to be loved. We may develop a 'false self' to present to the outside world, needing to hide the real self, which we feel to be unacceptable. So, if something good happens to us, it makes no difference to the unacceptable real self, and if something bad happens then it is further proof of our unacceptability.

Again, cultural voices impact these processes. The dismissive cultural voice which discourages us from thinking about our emotional life was also at work in our childhood, discouraging us from seeking help. We may have heard an injunction such as 'put on a brave face' or, less kindly, 'Don't be a cry-baby'. Perhaps particularly in the period of World War Two and soon afterwards, with so much suffering around, there was a feeling that emotional pain counted for little. We might recall being told 'There's no use crying over spilt milk' or, more cryptically, 'Worse things happen at sea'. These voices reinforced the idea that emotions are best dealt with by ignoring them.

Trauma

In addition to the effects on emotional development, there are voices that come as a direct result of trauma. Trauma is a complex issue and the experience of different kinds of traumas, such as bullying, physical abuse and sexual abuse, and in different contexts, leaves us with somewhat different messages about ourselves. But one common factor is that the experience of pain and distress being inflicted on us by a more powerful other can leave us with a message that our pain and our fear are not worth anything, and that our wishes are things to be ignored. This can lead to an internalized voice such as 'my feelings are not important' or, more simply, 'I am worthless', which may lead us to withdraw from interactions and relationships or not to protest if we experience further abuse later in life. It is also important to recognize that severe trauma can lead us to detach from our feelings (a process known as dissociation). This can make us feel 'broken' and confused, often with unpredictable emotional shifts. We may come to dismiss ourselves as 'damaged goods'.

Often, the experience of abuse is accompanied by powerlessness to seek help and sometimes by direct threats as to what will happen to us if we do. There is often a message, sometimes directly, that we deserve the distress that we are experiencing and that it is shameful. Again, this can add to an inner voice of worthlessness.

Our experience of childhood adversity is often complicated by other cultural voices about who we should and should not be. For men, there was (in many ways there still is) a very rigid idea of masculinity to live up to. Being 'emotional' was weak and pathetic. For women, there were lots of denigratory voices about girls and women's feebleness and incapacity, as well as ones strongly condemning any expression of sexuality, notably being pregnant or having a child outside of wedlock. There were racist cultural voices about, for instance, the stupidity of black people or the criminality of people from traveller communities. For anyone whose sexuality fell outside rigid cultural norms, there was intolerance, condemnation and criminalization. Experiencing mental health problems was seen as a moral weakness and worthy of ridicule. These voices can be internalized in their own right or reinforce and amplify internal voices of worthlessness that have come from our direct experience.

As we get towards old age, still further cultural voices come into play. These have to do with Western culture's view of older people. Research suggests that, while there are some positive stereotypes of older people, such as being seen as emotionally warm, there are many negative stereotypes (Hummert *et al*, 1994). Older people tend to be seen as being less capable, physically or intellectually, not as sexual or as sexually attractive, less creative and less able to learn new skills, more dependent, lonelier and more socially isolated. Cultural voices about aging are sometimes critical or derogatory, but also frequently mocking, which in some ways is even more undermining of our identity.

Moreover, while it has become much less acceptable to use stereotypes and make jokes about people based on their race or gender, older people are often seen as 'fair game', even among apparently progressive people. As political divisions between the generations have been emphasized in the UK, new age-related derogatory terms such as 'boomer' and 'gammon' have been coined and are seen as acceptable in many quarters.

In response to these voices, many people end up making jokes about themselves, such as talking about 'senior moments', and while this can be a way of taking control of the stereotype and making it less potent, it is also a sign of the way that the cultural voices can be internalized and potentially add to any existing negative voices about ourselves. If we already feel bad about the way that our life has gone, inhabiting a culture where we are seen as weak, incapable and 'past it' is only going to amplify the voice.

When we are faced with very negative ideas about ourselves, perhaps what we need is to find a different voice, which comes from a different story about ourselves and our life. This needs to be a story where we are the hero in our life; not necessarily in the sense of doing heroic deeds, but similar to the hero of a film, the story should be able to understand our choices and our reasons. I think it also needs to be a compassionate story, which recognizes that, being human, we will have weaknesses and make mistakes, which does not demand perfection but accepts us being 'good enough'. CAT therapy aims to help us to find such a story, but while can be easier to find this working together with a therapist, it is still helpful to think things through on our own. It is possible to find a compassionate story and a compassionate voice in conversation with ourselves.

Alice

To illustrate these ideas, I want to tell the story of a lady that I will call Alice. Because of the need for confidentiality, I did not want to take a real clinical example, so she is not a real person, but her story draws on the many stories I have had the privilege of hearing over the years.

She is a lady in her seventies who seeks help because of recurring depression and feeling that she has failed at everything she has done.

Alice grew up in Cambridgeshire in the 1950s. She was the second child but was much younger than her elder brother and never felt close to him. She described her mother and father as distant, strict and not physically affectionate. She realized as an adult that they were stressed by the effort of running a hotel which never seemed to make them much money. She felt they never had much time for her, or when she was honest, interest in her. She was an intelligent girl who liked reading but was shy. Despite her shyness, she did well at school, although she struggled to make friends. She remembered play being disapproved of at home; she loved to play with dolls, but she remembers being told that there were better things for her to do with her time. When out of school, she was expected to work at the hotel and was not allowed to bring friends home.

She did well enough in her exams to have the chance to apply to university, but her parents were not keen. They felt it was better to 'get her head down' and 'get a proper career'. She went into nursing. She did well in her career, becoming a ward manager, but found that it took a lot out of her and, as her career went on, she found she needed to take increasing time out with stress and depression.

She married but was left by her husband who met another woman when their daughter, Jenny, was two. She raised Jenny as a single parent. She spoke about how she loved her more than anything in the world and wanted her to have a happier life than Alice had, but struggled to express herself to Jenny and found herself being stricter than she wanted to be.

After her father died, her mother got dementia. Alice gave up her job to try to look after her, but she struggled to cope with her mother's increasing confusion and need for help. When her mother went into a home, she felt she had failed as a daughter.

Jenny has now moved away. They do not have a close relationship and Alice rarely sees her grandchildren. She does have a good friend from her nursing days but feels envious of the closer relationships that she has with her family. Alice feels ashamed of envying her friend.

The key to Alice finding a new story and a new voice to herself is understanding how hard it was for her as a child. The lack of emotional care and support she experienced made it difficult for her in several different ways. Both from her relationship with her mother and father and from the culture of the time, she internalized a voice along the lines of 'don't make a fuss' about her own emotions. Again, from the seeming lack of interest of her mother and father, she internalized a voice which said that her enjoyment was not important. This was amplified by a cultural voice that told her that girls and women should be 'caring' rather than 'selfish', and that it was not important for women to be educated.

She did not get the chance to learn to look after herself emotionally so she concentrated on caring for others, perhaps hoping that this would earn her love in return. Her lack of experience of a good caring relationship made it difficult for when she needed to look after first Jenny and then her mother, leading to outbursts of anger which made her feel like a failure. She had also internalized a critical voice that told her that her achievements were not worth anything and that she must always do better. This was amplified by the cultural voice which devalues caring work.

Despite all these difficulties, she had put enormous amounts of love and compassion into her role as a mother, in her role as a nurse and in caring for her mother. It is important for her to recognize how much she had given, how her compassion had kept her mother out of care for longer and given Jenny a much better start in life than she ever had.

In addition to the cultural voices that helped shape her childhood and her choices of roles, perhaps there is also a present-day voice telling us that the value of older women is in their relationships, particularly with children and grandchildren, and that they are failing if they do not have close family relationships or if they have negative feelings towards their friends.

If she was able to develop a more compassionate internal voice about her life and her achievements, she might be able to work on looking after herself emotionally. This might then lead to relationships such as with Jenny or her friend being easier to manage.

An exercise: Reflecting on your own life story

If this chapter has prompted you to reflect on your own life and any negative ideas you have about it, you may find the following exercise useful. It can be done in your mind but perhaps is more useful as a writing exercise. When answering the questions, it is important to try to hold onto a frame of mind which is sympathetic to yourself. It may help to imagine that you are writing through the eyes of someone who is sympathetic and not judgemental towards you. If you start it but are not in the right frame of mind, you could leave it to another time. If you are struggling to hold onto any sympathy, you might need to talk to someone else about the questions, perhaps a friend or a counsellor.

What did you find difficult as a child? In particular, what was difficult emotionally? Were there situations where you didn't know how to cope, or times when you were very afraid? It is important to try to acknowledge anything that made life more difficult. Try to ignore those cultural voices that tell you it was nothing.	
Were there any things about you, your thoughts and feelings that felt abnormal or shameful? This could include fears or wishes or desires or anything that made you feel different from other people.	
What voices did you hear about yourself – from parents and those around you? Think about how difficulties were responded to. Responses were most often well intentioned, but how helpful were they really?	

What voices did you hear about yourself from the world at large? Think about general cultural voices such as: 'Don't make a fuss', but also ones more particularly directed at you such as: Boys don't cry'. How did negative stereotypes or expectations about things such as your gender, sexuality, race or social class affect you?	
How did these experiences and voices affect the way that you felt about yourself and dealt with distress? What did you think about yourself and how did you cope with this?	
How did these struggles affect your relationships with others as you grew up? Were you confident in building friendships and relationships or did you avoid getting too close? Or did you seek out people to look after you or that you could look after? Perhaps you felt you had to hide your True Self and present only the part that felt 'acceptable'.	
How did these struggles affect your adult life? Think about relationships, education and career. Did they hold you back? Did you end up using coping strategies such as drinking, that caused more problems?	
How did any struggles in your life affect the way you thought about yourself? Did you end up feeling like you were useless or unlovable or a failure? Do you think that cultural voices about success and failure were part of this?	

If you experienced mental health problems or other adversity in your adult life, how did this affect the way that you felt about yourself? Again, think about the ideas you learned in your childhood and those of today.	
What did you achieve despite the difficulties? There are cultural voices that tell us not to acknowledge our achievements but to try to be generous to ourselves! Achievements are not usually about doing extraordinary things, they are often doing ordinary things in challenging circumstances.	
Who and what helped you to achieve what you achieved? Were there any supportive or sympathetic voices?	
What have you experienced getting older? How did this affect the way that you feel about yourself? Think about the positive and the negative. How have life and health changes impacted the way you feel about yourself? How have stereotypes about aging – positive and negative – affected you?	
Are there any particular voices, either from individuals or cultural voices, that make it hard for you to accept the way that your life has gone? Are there people you have been trying to please? Or standards that you are under pressure to live up to? Do you need to keep pushing yourself in this way?	

If you could go back and talk to your younger self with the benefit of experience – what would you say? Think about what life has taught you about what is important and what isn't.	
What will help you find acceptance of yourself and your life going forwards? This is a tough one – it may take time to develop new perspectives and work towards acceptance.	

As a guide, I have imagined some answers that Alice might have given in the table below.

What did you find difficult as a child? In particular, what was difficult emotionally? Were there situations where you didn't know how to cope, or times when you were very afraid? It is important to try to acknowledge anything that made life more difficult. Try to ignore those cultural voices that tell you it was nothing.	My mum and dad provided for me and looked after me, but they weren't warm people. They were always so busy. I would cry on my own because it felt like there was no one to turn to.
Were there any things about you, your thoughts and feelings that felt abnormal or shameful? This could include fears or wishes or desires or anything that made you feel different from other people.	I felt like I was always a baby with babyish thoughts and feelings. I kept them to myself.
What voices did you hear about yourself – from parents and those around you? Think about how difficulties were responded to. Responses were most often well intentioned, but how helpful were they really?	I felt like my parents were never very interested in me, as if they were saying I wasn't worth bothering with.

What voices did you hear about yourself from the world at large? Think about general cultural voices such as: 'Don't make a fuss', but also ones more particularly directed at you such as: Boys don't cry'. How did negative stereotypes or expectations about things such as your gender, sexuality, race or social class affect you?	I feel like girls of my generation weren't supposed to want anything, just be sensible and practical. You had to 'smile and get on with it'.
How did these experiences and voices affect the way that you felt about yourself and dealt with distress? What did you think about yourself and how did you cope with this?	I felt like I wasn't worth a whole lot. I should just put my head down and get on with it.
How did these struggles affect your relationships with others as you grew up? Were you confident in building friendships and relationships or did you avoid getting too close? Or did you seek out people to look after you or that you could look after? Perhaps you felt you had to hide your True Self and present only the part that felt 'acceptable'.	I didn't make friends as I was growing up. I never thought people would be bothered with me unless they needed me to do something for them.
How did these struggles affect your adult life? Think about relationships, education and career. Did they hold you back? Did you end up using coping strategies such as drinking, that caused more problems?	I wanted to go to university but didn't feel like they took my sort of person. I don't regret being a nurse, but I wonder if I could have been something else. If I'm honest I didn't make a good choice of husband. I made do. I just couldn't believe anyone would really care about me.

How did any struggles in your life affect the way you thought about yourself? Did you end up feeling like you were useless or unlovable or a failure? Do you think that cultural voices about success and failure were part of this?	I loved Jenny so much. She was my little miracle, but she was so demanding. I ended up shouting at her and feeling like an awful mum. I felt like I'd failed as a mother and then failed again when Mum got dementia.
If you experienced mental health problems or other adversity in your adult life, how did this affect the way that you felt about yourself? Again, think about the ideas you learned in your childhood and those of today.	It was awful when I couldn't work because of depression. I thought I was a self-indulgent waste of space. I can see now that I couldn't help it, but it felt awful.
What did you achieve despite the difficulties? There are cultural voices that tell us not to acknowledge our achievements but to try to be generous to ourselves! Achievements are not usually about doing extraordinary things, they are often doing ordinary things in challenging circumstances.	I suppose I did OK in my job. Sometimes the ward was running smoothly and I felt like I could cope with anything. And I did OK with Jenny really, all on my own. She's turned out well even if I wish I saw a bit more of her.
Who and what helped you to achieve what you achieved? Were there any supportive or sympathetic voices?	Rita, my old boss, was great when I was flapping. She would say to me 'You can only do what you can'. And sometimes I found myself talking to her about Jenny. She didn't give me advice always, but I just felt a bit less alone with it.

What have you experienced getting older? How did this affect the way that you feel about yourself? Think about the positive and the negative. How have life and health changes impacted the way you feel about yourself? How have stereotypes about aging – positive and negative – affected you?	I don't like getting older. I can sometimes walk down the street and feel completely invisible, and it's not easy when you have more time but don't have enough money to enjoy it. I feel lonely sometimes. I feel like you're supposed to be playing happy families when you're my age and it's not easy with Jenny being so distant and so busy. I feel sad and I think 'You can't be bothered either'.
Are there any particular voices, either from individuals or cultural voices, that make it hard for you to accept the way that your life has gone? Are there people you have been trying to please? Or standards that you are under pressure to live up to? Do you need to keep pushing yourself in this way?	I think I was trying to get everything right – I think maybe I was trying to get Mum and Dad to notice me for once, to be proud of me. But that was never going to happen.
If you could go back and talk to your younger self with the benefit of experience – what would you say? Think about what life has taught you about what is important and what isn't.	I'd say to myself 'Do that University application, give it a go. If it doesn't work out, you can try something else later.'
What will help you find acceptance of yourself and your life going forwards? This is a tough one – it may take time to develop new perspectives and work towards acceptance.	I suppose when I look back on my life, I didn't really do so bad. I got through and tried to take care of people. I have to try to remember Rita – 'You can only do what you can'.

Summary

I hope that reflecting on these questions is helpful. However, it is important to recognize that cultural voices about success and failure and what it is to be a good or bad person are powerful things. Talking it through with another person, whether a friend or a counsellor or therapist, may make it easier. I often think that the people who cope best with the trials of living and getting older are those (usually by luck) who are part of a family or a group who provide more supportive or compassionate voices to speak against the criticism and judgement of our wider culture. In an ideal world, we would all find ourselves such a group, or be able to build a group – a 'microculture' that is able to offer support and acceptance. However, in the real world we often have to think it through for ourselves. If that is what you are doing, good luck! I hope that you are able to use the voices of this chapter and this book to help you find a better and a kinder voice with which to speak to yourself.

Chapter 5: Who am I really? A CAT reflection on retirement

Henrietta Batchelor

No one lives his life.

Disguised since childhood,
haphazardly assembled
from voices and fears and little pleasures,
we come of age as masks.
Our true face never speaks.
Somewhere there must be storehouses
where all these lives are laid away
like suits of armor or old carriages
or clothes hanging limply on the walls.
Maybe all the paths lead there,
to the repository of unlived things.

(Rainer Maria Rilke, 1905)

Introduction

When I was in my early fifties, a group of us, members of a North East of England psychology Special Interest Group, asked Joyce McDougal, a well-regarded New Zealand-French psychoanalyst (Theatres of Mind, 1982, Theatres of the Body, 1989) to come and speak to our group. She was in her late seventies, attractive, witty, intelligent, generous and warm. We were all entranced not only by her presentation but also by her personality. We all said that this is how we would like to be by the time we were approaching our own eightieth birthdays. As I have got older and nearer to retirement age, I have often thought of Joyce, but I am also rather haunted by another spectre – that of an aging psychotherapist, not keeping up with current research, and working on well past their sell-by date. It has happened. Freud worked into his eighties, notwithstanding his struggle with a painful oral cancer which made it difficult to speak and was reportedly so malodourous that even his dog left the room (Gay,1988).

In CAT, we might represent this dilemma as: *either* admired and desired *or* despairing and deluded (see Chapter 2). The common-sense way out of this dilemma (the 'exit', in CAT terms) would be to find a role that was at neither extreme but somewhere in the middle. However, drawing on clinical and personal experience, basing your life on any *role* without first working out the wishes, needs and values that underpin such a role may be an unproductive strategy.

This chapter considers the meaning of work in our lives and what might be gained and/or lost in retirement, drawing on research and general psychological theories. For many of us, retirement is a step-change, a whole or partial change of role and, like other life changes, such as leaving home or having a baby, deserves the same kind of consideration and thought. Our new 'way of being' may not be quite how we imagined it to be, but it can be a meaningful and productive post-career move, depending on how we manage this transition. This awareness may be sharpened by the perceived and actual proximity of death. In contrast to earlier life changes, there are few 'second chances' for this phase of life. Whether welcomed or dreaded, retirement is a life-stage transition which needs to be accommodated. There may be feelings of loss and regret but also more positive emotions – including relief at having more time at one's disposal and excitement about exploring new interests. Our relationship with institutions and workplace settings is also considered and how letting go of work not only impacts individuals but relationships as well. It is suggested that the psychological task is to understand and nurture what is beneath our social and work personas so that the 'here and now' of a post-work life can be truly explored in an authentic way. These ideas will be explored through a variety of psychological models, along with CAT understandings through vignettes and clinical examples together with potential 'exits' – strategies which may be helpful when facilitating this experience.

Retirement and later life

The age at which people can receive their state pension in the UK is currently sixty-six. This will gradually increase from May 2026. Given documented increases in life expectancy, depending on socioeconomic and health inequalities, many people can expect to live a significant length of their life beyond this 'retirement age'. The ONS (2022) states that a record number of over sixty-fives are currently in work – at the time of the survey, close to 1.5 million. This increase is driven by part-time workers with most over sixty-fives working between sixteen and thirty hours per week. Reasons vary and include the need for income over and above work or statutory pensions, or the need by employers to retain expertise, or because retirees feel that they have 'more to give' to their workplace. Analysis is complicated by the varying terms in which post-full-time workers are described. Some are described as in 'phased retirement', or in 'partial employment', others in 'bridge employment' (a job between full-time work and retirement), and others may be self-employed in a job connected or quite different from their recent work role. But clearly, a significant proportion of those of us over sixty-fives are not fully retired.

However much retirement has been considered in advance, the loss of paid work may feel subject to societal pressures which privilege youth and material success. However, others propose that retirement can be seen not as a loss but as another active stage in our lives. Wang (2014, p313) describes retirement as 'a career opportunity stage… not a career exit but a late career development'. Some retirees would not identify with the word 'loss' and feel that they can embrace letting go of formal work enthusiastically. Some people may have a hobby or interest that can take the place of paid employment. Others may phase themselves out of work feeling that letting go gradually is the right way for them. And some may branch out into self-employment.

But many retirees may feel lost, at least in the short term. And, as noted above, a further complicating factor is that this new phase of life is likely to coincide with being older. This distinguishes retirement from other life-stage transitions as it also may well overlap with the onset of illness, either one's own or that of a partner or parent – or with other life changes such as bereavement or the need to offer childcare to a younger generation. This means that planning a new and rewarding life for oneself can be complicated.

Exercise

Thinking about your own experiences:

- Have you retired from formal work completely or partially?
- Did you have a choice about how this came about or was it driven by other factors?
- What were your feelings as you approached this transition?
- What are the negative aspects of retirement?
- What are the opportunities?
- What do you regret?
- What will be a relief?

The meaning of work in our lives

We bring into adult life the influences of our genetic makeup and our childhood experiences. Many psychological therapists including Jung (Stevens, 1994) and Erikson (1950) believed that personal growth is lifelong and that work is a place which may be, in an enriching situation, challenging and supportive of continuing personal growth. Mattinson (1988) describes how work provides the following:

- A time structure.
- Shared experiences outside the family.
- Linkage to goals and purposes outside a person's ambitions.
- Identity and status.
- Purposeful activity.
- A satisfaction of unconscious needs – see section below.

Many of us would also say that the financial recompense of work is not only important because it buys things, but that it also augments our sense of self-worth.

Figure 5.1: Maslow's Hierarchy of Needs

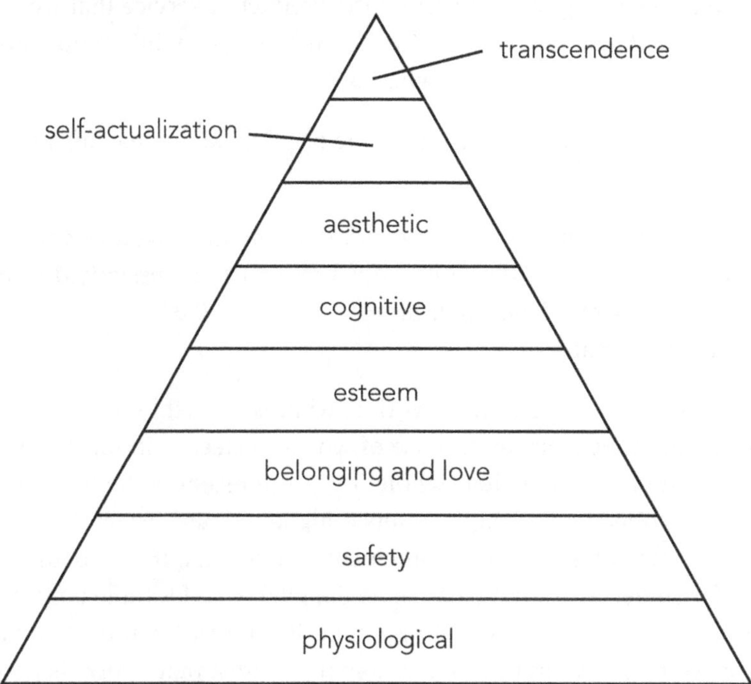

Considering Maslow's Hierarchy of Needs (1943) (Figure 5.1), work may satisfy on a number of levels – from the individual through to the organizational, as well as societal and cultural. Those employed by organizations may feel that work confers the safety of a predictable income and a sense of belonging. Companies build on this need to belong as it can promote a sense of well-being and works to retain staff. Most companies have 'mission statements' or use concepts like 'brand' and 'brand loyalty'. In her book *Willing Slaves: How overwork culture is ruling our lives* (2004), Madeline Bunting argues that we can be exploited by large organizations. The workforce, she argues, is eager for wealth and satisfaction, but instead hard work has brought worry, illness, and in some cases poverty and debt. Brand loyalty gives the illusion that the company is bringing some kind of meaning into people's lives. For example, on their website, Asda, a UK-based supermarket describes the 'Asda Family':

> '...*our colleagues are the heroes, and they have always made Asda special. Every one of us shapes the character of this company.*'

All of us who have worked in big institutions are familiar with a special sort of language that grows up around the product or service that we sell or provide. This reinforces the 'brand' as there is an 'in' group who understand it and an 'out' group who don't.

Thus, leaving an organization is, for some people, akin to leaving a family. As one person put it:

> '*You lose a community and along with it a common language and shared understanding of complex topics in a narrow, specialized field that probably won't have application in your new life.*'
> (Private conversation)

For many, across many cultures, work is what is valued by society and, to that extent, affects our own sense of worth ('esteem', in Maslow's terms). For some, work is their whole life. More recently, the 'overwork culture', described by Bunting, confers a higher status – to work all hours with high stress, however much complained about, is a badge of honour for some. 'Work-life balance' is dangled as a desirable concept but for many it doesn't really gain traction. But for those of us who are older, as we retire, we have to grapple with the idea that 'work' is good and 'not-work' is less desirable. We may be faced with others asking the unthinking question: 'What do you *do* now?' as if *doing something* is good, and *not doing* [work] diminishes us in some way. Chapter 2 explains a CAT way of understanding this phenomenon. How others or an outside environment relate to us, becomes part of our own 'self-to-self' inner conversation. So, if it is only work that speaks to us about our value and usefulness (*valuing* making us feel *valued and needed*), then the absence of work may make us feel irrelevant (*dismissing* in relation to *irrelevant and past it*) – see Figure 5.2. We may need to unpick what it is about work that has enriched us, and, as we stop work, take some of those attributes into an 'after-work' life. We may have to reimagine our own priorities and values and be robust in challenging negative views of retirement from the environment around us. Small things may become important as opposed to large-scale grand projects.

Figure 5.2: Adjustment to retirement

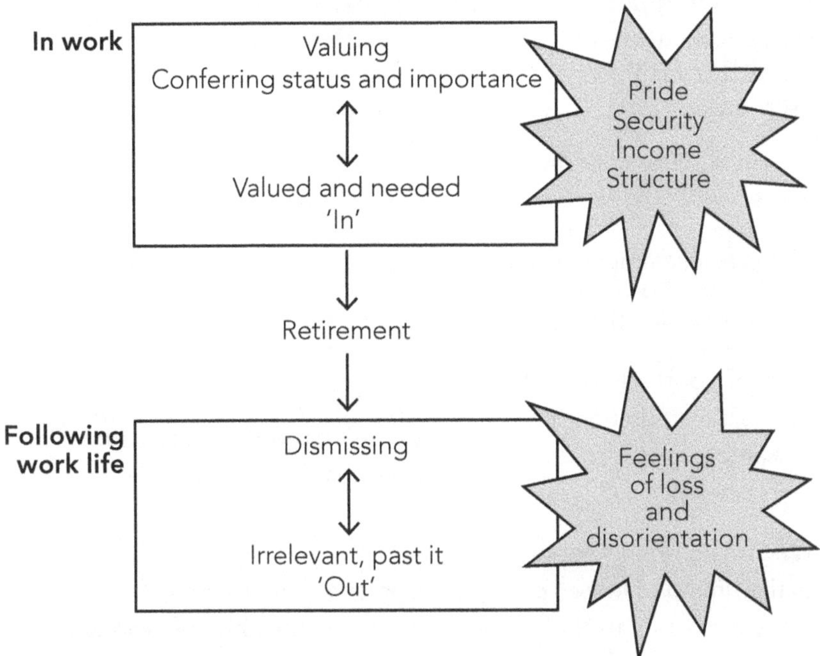

Inevitably, some of us will adjust to retirement – or even partial retirement – better than others. Some of the attributes of retirees that affect the transition to retirement are listed by Wang (2014) in Table 5.1.

Exercise

As you read through the list in Table 5.1, tick those that apply to you from both columns. This may help you to understand your thoughts and feelings after (or as you approach) retirement and identify those areas over which you might have some control. For instance, if you have few or no hobbies, are there things that you have always wanted to do or would like to do now?

Table 5.1: Factors in transitioning to retirement	
Positive indicators of a smooth transition to retirement	**Negative indicators of a more problematic adjustment to retirement**
Having a number of non-work hobbies.	Few outside work interests.
Less social investment in work.	High identification with work role.
Having a flexible attitude.	Rigid thinking.
History of good adjustment to previous life-stage transitions (for example, going to university, having a baby).	Poorer adjustment to life-stage transitions and/or associations with previous difficult events.
Having an active engagement with the timing of retirement, realistic expectations and planning ahead for this change of lifestyle.	Unplanned retirement or low engagement with the process, including being forced to retire.
Having enough money for the desired post-work lifestyle.	Restricted finances.
Good mental and physical health.	Poor mental or physical health.
A happy relationship.	Less harmonious relationships, or single or widowed.
Lower number of dependents.	Dependents needing support.

Some of the attributes in Table 5.1 are perhaps predictable. Less obvious are other features influencing adjustment. Houlfort *et al* (2015) look at the role that passion plays in people's employment. The authors describe is that, 'harmonious passion for work predicts good psychological adjustment in retirement' and, conversely, 'obsessive passion for work' leads to poorer adjustment in retirement. According to Wang (2014), high stress levels – 'burn out' – at work do not correlate well with a new post-work life.

He suggests that there may be some short-term relief, but in the longer term, individuals are likely to fare less well. No reason is suggested but Figure 5.3 describes a situation in reciprocal role terms. Retrospectively, a retiree may have to accommodate a legacy of anger and a history of feeling powerless and without agency. One of the main factors positively influencing a productive retirement is to proactively take control of a new phase of life so this may be the new challenge. Understanding the contextual and relational dynamics at play here can help to make sense of such feelings and find ways to manage them going forwards.

Case study: Julie

Julie was referred to an older adult psychology service by her GP, experiencing acute anxiety and low mood. She had worked part time for twenty-five years for a small building firm as their bookkeeper. At first, she had enjoyed the work, but as the firm took on more business her workload grew exponentially but without any pay increase. For the last five years of her working life, she was exhausted and demoralized and counted the days to her retirement. On her last day, she learned that her role would be replaced with a chartered accountant who would work full-time and would be paid considerably more than her.

Julie was brought up in a family who, although not well off, cared for her material needs, but whose mantra was 'just get on with it, there's no point in complaining'. Initially, Julie felt relief that she no longer had to face the daily grind of work. But she gradually became depressed and at times so anxious that it was difficult to leave the house. Her CAT therapist helped her unpack the events of her working life, noting how she felt that her loyalty to the firm, especially in the early days when she felt she had a real role in keeping it going, had been betrayed by their exploitation of her goodwill. As the firm grew, she felt that new managers had 'treated her like dirt' and she wished she had been able to stand up to them. Together, she and her therapist drew a map that captured how she felt. Although she could identify anger with her employers, it also made her feel anxious and panicky and out of control. One of the things that helped her most was to write a 'no send' letter to the managers that expressed her feelings and – as she put it – 'got things out of her system'.

Figure 5.3: Stress and retirement – Julie's map

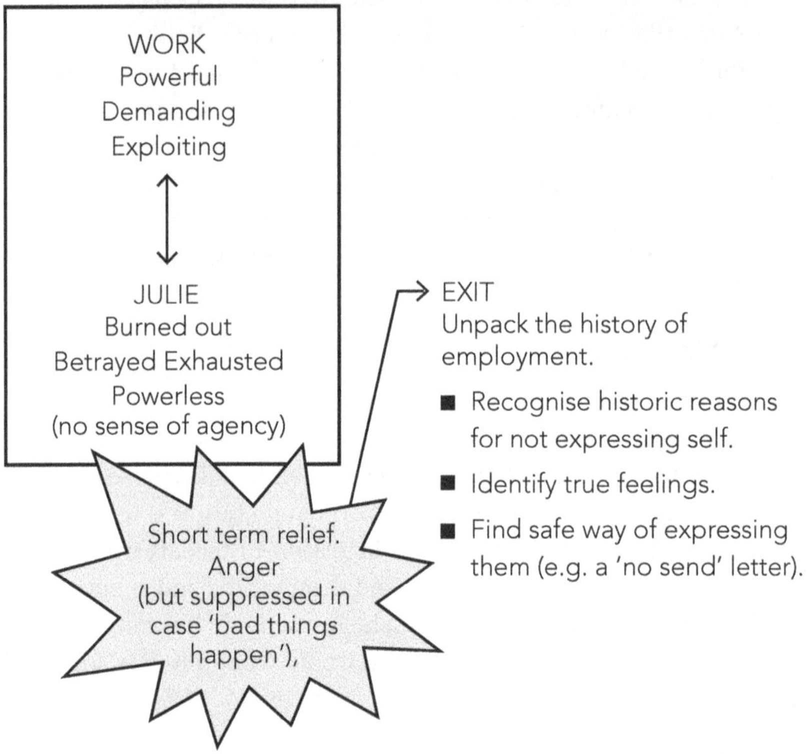

The impact of health and gender on retirement

A history of unemployment, especially if just before retirement, does not bode well for retirement (Wang, 2014). If unemployment has been a result of long-term sick leave, individuals may struggle to come to terms with not only their poor health, but also the new status quo.

Despite aspirations towards gender equality, the majority of women take on a larger share of domestic and care work in addition to managing any formal employment (Criado Perez, 2019). Anecdotally, women are supposed to fare better in retirement than men, perhaps because the flexibility in juggling tasks means that they are better able to adjust to a new post-work phase of life. Surprisingly few studies have explored the influence of gender on psychological well-being in retirement. Richardson & Kilty (2008) measured psychological symptoms of distress pre-retirement, again at six months, and then a year later. They found that women expressed more anxiety after retirement. Men were more likely to express their distress somatically. One analysis (Peltier *et al*, 2020) states that the use of alcohol has increased in the last two decades in adults over sixty, and especially so among women, along with increased rates of binge drinking. This is, of course, the age when many are planning to retire or have retired, and may be one way of coping with this major life change. Excessive drinking is obviously not healthy, but it also contributes to falls and other drink-related injuries and conditions.

Kubicek *et al* (2011) also suggest that some factors for retirement satisfaction are different for men and women – men's well-being is more likely to be positively influenced by financial assets, while women are more concerned with social relationships. It certainly appears that women save less than men for this phase of life (Cribb *et al*, 2023) and there is a significant gender gap in pensions, with men having 25% on average more than women (OECD, 2020). One in four older women workers are ineligible for automatic workplace pension enrolment because they work part time (Centre for Ageing Better, 2022). Financial security is obviously an important factor in post-retirement well-being, particularly if a pension is not buttressed by that of a partner.

Zelenski (2022) – like Mattinson (1988), above – summarizes it well when he writes that work provides a structure, routine, community and purpose in life, and this needs to be transposed into retirement. He suggests that, in retirement, we now need to 'dream on [our] own, plan on [our]own and make decisions on [our] own'. To some, this must seem like utter bliss, to others, daunting in the extreme, and to some of us a bit of both!

The dynamics of institutions and our connection with them

Figure 5.2 suggests that it might be a loss to retire from a post that confers value and importance, and Figure 5.3 that it is a relief (at least initially) to get out of a job where you have become burnt out. In this section, I consider what we may have projected (where someone unconsciously attributes their thoughts, feelings, or behaviours to another person/people) onto institutions and the challenge we face to our integrity when we retire.

In her book *Work, Love and Marriage* (1988), Janet Mattinson likens the individual's relationship with work to that between partners in marriage or a committed relationship. Sometimes, the relationship with the institution or organization can feel like that of a parent to a child. The division of roles can feel benign at times: in CAT, we might say that an institution is *caring* in relation to which an individual feels *cared for and appreciated* (as in a good-enough relationship between parent and child). Sometimes, though, the reverse is true, and an organization is all-powerful and in relation to this an individual may feel *crushed,* as if their life is not their own.

Mattinson suggests that we can project onto our work – or attribute to an employing institution – aspects of ourselves which we may not like or may not take responsibility for. She is saying that this is similar to what happens between partners in long-term relationships. So, for example, one partner may be more familiar with overt expressions of anger while their partner is afraid of being expressive in this way. By withdrawing from disagreements such that the first partner becomes enraged, the second partner may be *splitting off* a part of themselves (the capacity for expressing anger) and *projecting* it onto the other who then acts it out. So, to return to the work example above, an individual may project power and control onto the employing institution uncomfortable with or unaware of his or her own agency and personal power. Regaining autotomy in this instance may be one of the challenges of retirement. Or where the institution takes care of many of an individual's needs, on leaving the place or work that person needs to think through the care they may need to give themselves.

Clearly then, in retirement, these states of mind need to be re-introjected (taken back into the self). Henry Dicks (1967), an American psychoanalyst, suggests that part of the reason couples are attracted is that, at an unconscious level, they sense the need and also the capacity for this kind of projective 'economy'. Mattinson extends this idea to explore why some jobs have a particular appeal for us: there may be an unconscious attraction to a particular profession, particularly if this is vocational. Psychotherapists, nurses and social doctors may, by caring for others, meet a need in themselves. Accountants may enjoy a feeling of order that was perhaps missing from their early lives, prison officers may be attracted to a sense of control not there for them as young people. It follows, then, that, just as divorced or widowed partners experience intense emotions following the end of a relationship, so too the end of a career can elicit similar distress. It is not just the grief of loss in each case, but also the psychological need to re-integrate into the self that which has been projected onto the other or onto work.

Exercise

Think about the following questions and write down your response:

- What needs did your work fulfil?
- In retiring, will some or all of these needs go unmet?
- Or are there other ways to meet these?

Case study: Ryan

Ryan was referred to the army psychology service for Cognitive Analytic Therapy following an episode in which he had got into a fight with another soldier after excessive drinking. He was approaching retirement from the army, which had been planned when this incident happened. He had attended 'Resettlement Classes' provided by the army to help prepare him for his new life on 'Civvy Street'. He lived with his wife in army quarters and had some practical ideas for an active retirement. As the date for retirement approached, his mental health deteriorated and he described how his anger was often directed at his wife. Drinking numbed the feelings of shame arising from his loss of control. In discussion with his therapist, he described a fractured upbringing, in and out of care because of his mother's alcoholism and his father's violent behaviour towards his wife and children. Ryan was a wild child, often truanting from school and involved in petty crime. When his social worker suggested he join the army as a young 18-year-old recruit, Ryan was attracted to the opportunities for sport and adventure. Less conscious, perhaps, was that the army was a surrogate family that could provide structure, discipline and containment. In so far as he saw active duty, his aggression was channelled into army manoeuvres. Unconsciously, the army not only provided for his basic needs but also enabled Ryan to project his aggression safely onto the service. The prospect of retirement was terrifying: consciously, Ryan was ready to leave the army and live 'outside the wire'. Unconsciously, he feared losing control of the anger he felt which was triggered by any situation that reminded him of his childhood loss of security. Ryan had some reservations about the value of talking therapy. However, he felt that for the first time someone – his therapist – took his early deprivation seriously. He recognized the parallel between his current situation of losing his 'army family' with the traumatic memories of being removed from home and taken into care. As he became more able to separate past from present, Ryan recognized that he was no longer the troubled, out-of-control and immature boy who had no one to turn to – in contrast, he was a well-regarded and skilled adult, who had had a good work record and who was proud of the security he had given to his family. With the help of his therapist, he learned strategies to contain and manage his anger, just as the army had a professional structure and discipline for the use of force. The ones he found most useful are included on the map shown in Figure 5.4.

Figure 5.4: Ryan's personality structure

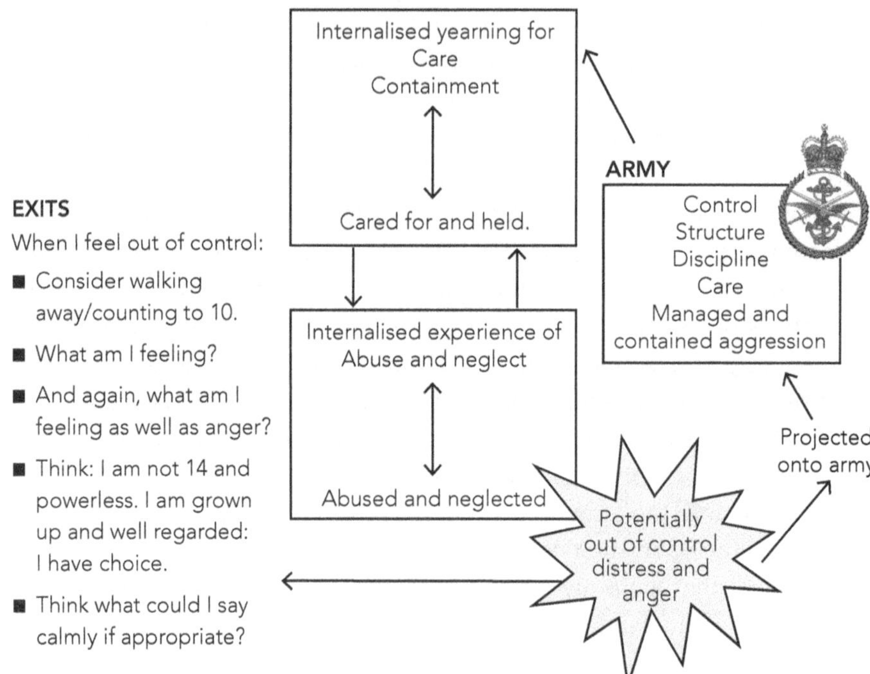

Work as an attachment, retirement as a loss of this attachment

The seeking and maintaining of a work role that provides structure, meaning and identity is likely to be experienced as an attachment. So even when retirement is experienced as a positive move, it is nevertheless a change, and to this extent can evoke several emotions akin to those experienced in grief (Bowlby, 1979). Thus, we would expect individuals to experience numbness, a yearning for what is lost, sadness, anger and disorientation. There are often other losses, too – relationships with other workers, pride in and respect for what one has achieved, social relationships, the status of a role at work, and sometimes the perks of a job such as a secretary or a company car. And, of course, money – both real pay and as a symbol of worth.

> 'Some weeks after I retired, I began to experience severe chest pains and was so worried I called an ambulance. The doctor explained that I was experiencing acute anxiety. On reflection, this made me think what a big deal it was leaving work. It was a routine, and although I made decisions about strategy and safety, in a way I didn't make any macro decisions – work was just decided for me. I planned to retire, but freedom from work was too much, boundless really… I think this is what caused the anxiety. I miss colleagues with whom I went through really difficult times. We shared both the adrenaline rush, the drama of rescuing, the shared memories… It was never dull. I am not one for talking about my feelings but I was amazed at how tearful I was. Retiring was like losing an old friend… I couldn't concentrate for months; I couldn't just get on with my new life.'
>
> (Private conversation with a retired fireman.)

In practice, life transitions are complex. Multiple inter-related transitions may occur concurrently or in succession. Retirement is a transition more likely to happen to older people and thus it is expected that other life changes may occur simultaneously. It is not uncommon for retirees to find themselves becoming carers just when they may have expected to have less responsibility. They may find themselves needed as grandparents, or to look after their own aging parents, or becoming responsible for a partner who becomes ill and dependent. And, of course, older may mean less physically resilient, so retirement plans are tempered by one's state of health.

Taking all of these factors into account, retirement as a life-stage transition needs to be accommodated, and this can be challenging, even if it is expected. However, for some people, retirement is enforced earlier than planned. Companies restructure and let part of their workforce go. Individuals decide to leave – or perhaps feel forced to leave – because of difficult workplace situations, such as bullying. Others retire on grounds of ill-health. All this impacts individuals but also their families, with implications for their security and well-being. These factors complicate coming to terms with letting go of paid employment. In relational terms, it may be helpful to draw out and name the dynamics so that the emotional reaction makes more sense. It is also important to note whether such a dynamic has been experienced as a child or young adult, in which case the intensity of the emotion may be more acute.

Positive emotions may arise from retirement, too: some report relief, others excitement and a sense of freedom, feeling released to 'to do their own thing'. A article in *The Guardian* (Dodd, 2018) titled 'Life keeps evolving', challenges some of the myths surrounding retirement. It exhorts us to challenge ageism as it 'eats into self-esteem'. Importantly, this article highlights that older age is a vast span of years, not static, but a chance to grow and develop in new ways.

A collapse of identity

Those at risk of a difficult transition into retirement are those for whom 'almost all their lives the fact of going to work was ... the key to [their] social legitimacy' (Osborne, 2009). The following quotes from retirees illustrate this crisis. For instance:

> '*Who am I apart from the roles I have been playing – some of them good, productive and consistent with my inner values and some not?*' (Hollis, 2006)

Or John Browne, CEO of BP, whose voluntary retirement was complicated by being 'outed' by a Sunday tabloid (Segalov, 2022):

> '[When you work for a big company] *there are all sorts of people looking after you and doing things for you. Then you are all alone. I had no secretary, no staff, no support. I had to build that for myself.*'

A CAT psychotherapist who held a senior role in a big NHS Trust describes how, even when retirement has been anticipated, the reality can come as a shock:

> '*...a* [reciprocal] *role collapse. One moment I was a valued member of a big community whose advice was sought and had so many things to do. And then... all that went.*' (Private conversation)

While acceptance of retirement needs to involve the consideration of what has been lost and gained, these quotes show that, for many people, the most profound feeling is that of a loss of identity or role. The more the individual has invested in work, the more acute this feeling may be. Who am I really if not an employee/director of a big company or a fireman/electrician/doctor/nurse etc?

Donald Winnicott, a psychiatrist and psychoanalyst working in the middle of the last century (Winnicott, 1960), addressed this question. As a child grows, inevitably they need to adapt socially to the outside world, which may mean becoming what their parents, schools and workplace require of them. He coined the idea of a 'True and False Self' – the former being the essential, uninfluenced and free self and the latter being the child and adult that has adapted to the society around them. There can be a healthy balance between the persona conferred on us by work and the essential self that resides outside of employment. However, if the only thing that 'feeds' self-esteem is the money, status, preoccupation etc. of a work role, and the inner self is neglected, then retirement is going to be a challenging time.

Returning to Erik Erikson (see Chapter 1), the task of the first of the older adult stages, relating to the dichotomous pair 'generativity and despair' (attained, according to Erikson, between fifty and seventy years), relates to an individual's need to give back skills and experience to a younger generation. This would certainly include children and younger members of a community, but one interpretation of this is a social one: for potential retirees to hand on the baton of their experience to a younger generation. In social terms, perhaps the older generation does need to step away from a job, perhaps held for many years, in order to give a younger generation a chance to make their contribution. This would represent 'care' of both a younger generation but also 'care' of insight and experience gained in a working life.

The final stage of a person's life is to gain psychological integrity and it is worth quoting a passage from *Childhood and Society* (Erikson, 1950) to explain what is meant by this:

> *'It is the acceptance of one's one and only life cycle as something that had to be and that, by necessity, permitted of no substitutions: it thus means a new, a different love of one's parents. It is a comradeship with the ordering ways of distant times and different pursuits, as expressed in the simple products and sayings of such times and pursuits.... [T]he possessor of integrity is ready to defend the dignity of his own lifestyle against all physical and economic threats. For he knows that an individual life is the accidental coincidence of but one life cycle with but one segment of history...'*

Erikson is suggesting that, in the context of a working life, we need to come to terms with regrets and disappointments, 'the roads less travelled', so that there is a sense of closure and completeness, and we can accept death without fear. This, he suggests, leads to wisdom.

But given so many people faced with retirement feel that their very identity is on the line, it is worth revisiting Erikson's earlier stage, normally pertaining to adolescents. He calls this: Identity vs Role Confusion (desired outcome: Fidelity). The adolescent's task is to find a route to separation-individuation by becoming their authentic self (their 'True Self' in Winnicott's terms) neither a product of their parents' wishes and values nor overinfluenced by society. The outcome 'Fidelity' refers to being true or faithful to oneself. So, as we leave work, the question is: are we defined by work, its culture and our role within it, or do we have enough of our True Self as opposed to being falsely defined? We might want to ask what has been lost as we have compliantly adapted to a work persona. The poem by Rilke at the beginning of the chapter suggests that there may be 'storehouses' of hidden or unexplored lives. There are opportunities offered by the transition to a post-work stage of life, notably to find that which may have been overlooked or lost on the journey to making an 'honest crust'. We will reflect on this some more below, in the section 'Going forwards: what helps?'

Exercise

- What hobbies, interests and activities have been lost as a result of being employed?
- What might you pick up again when you have more time?

'For better or for worse but not for lunch': the impact of retirement on relationships

Self-evidently, leaving work means that it is likely that an individual will spend more time at home. For many couples, this is something that is positively anticipated. But time spent together increases the intimacy of a relationship and also, therefore, the potential for conflict. There is of course no right answer for how much time should be spent together; this is a matter for each couple – communication is key. Long-held patterns of communication – or miscommunication – may come to the fore for the first time, alongside challenges to previously held roles, for example, who does what jobs around the home, who manages the money, and so on. Renegotiating relational roles with partners, family members and friends is all part of this transition. Such changes can be made easier by having a better sense of your own part in the relational 'dance'.

Case study: Marion and Jack

Marion looked forward to Jack's retirement, anticipating that they would spend more time together, he would be less preoccupied with work, and that they would have enough money and time to travel now he was retired and the children had left home. She had retired a few years earlier. But this was not Jack's plan. He missed the stimulus of work and enrolled on a university course, which meant he spent time away from home and, while he enjoyed the company of a younger generation of students, he was upset and angered that his wife accused him of excluding her and finding other people more interesting.

Neither Marion nor Jack had communicated their needs to one another, a long-held pattern within their relationship but without major issue for the most part in their earlier years. For them, as for many of us, work lulls us into a predictable status quo and, of course, retirement or even partial retirement is a step-change. In discussion with their therapist, this couple could discuss this problem, but it revealed deeper issues regarding closeness and exclusion that had been masked by the need for them to go to work. Their therapist asked them to complete the exercise illustrated below. Both were surprised to understand how their expectations differed. Jack worried that, having freedom from the commitment of work, he did not want to be 'told' how to spend his leisure time. Marion felt this was a deeply unfair caricature of her as controlling and bossy. In CAT terms, they agreed that they enacted a *perceived* reciprocal role of 'controlling and bossy' to 'crushed and wanting to bolt for freedom'. The couple's therapist was intrigued to know more about what 'control' and 'being restricted' meant to this couple. Marion and Jack came to see that Jack had a deep fear of control as he felt his own father had been emasculated by a domineering mother, and Marion had always been afraid of losing 'her man', having grown up with a philandering father whose infidelities impacted the whole family. Their shared fear was that partners could not be trusted to be equal companions and lovers, *and* have their individual lives. Work had acted as an intimacy regulator for many years, and while this honest exchange of feelings was painful, this 'crunch point' was an opportunity for a better mutual understanding and growth as a couple. As the couple worked through their difficulties, they were better able to negotiate with one another without feeling threatened. One strategy ('exit' in CAT terms) that was helpful was for each to distinguish between what went on in the past and to approach their own present and future proactively and assertively. As their anxiety was contained in therapy, they came to see that there was plenty of time for individual activities as well as planning exciting joint ventures. And, as their couple relationship grew, so trust deepened and the spectre of infidelity diminished.

The poet Kahlil Gibran (1923) has some wise advice written in a passage from *The Prophet*, often read at weddings:

> *Let there be spaces in your togetherness.*
> *And let the winds of the heavens dance between you.*
> *Love one another but make not a bond of love...*

Exercise

Draw two sets of two overlapping circles. The first set is for pre-retirement, the second to your expectation of how life might be after retirement. For each pair, label one of the circles 'Partner's time alone', and the other 'My time alone', and, where the two circles intersect, 'Our time together'. This is an exercise best done together for ease of communication.

When you have done this:

- Consider what activities would you like to do on your own.
- What would you like to do together?

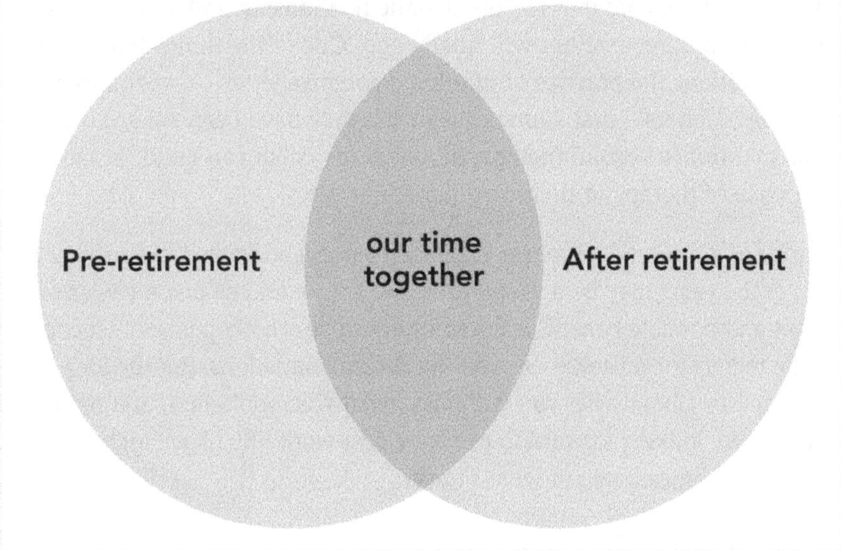

While there is a loneliness about being in an unhappy marriage, single men and women are particularly at risk of loneliness following any loss – for example, the loss of a partner or the loss of good health. So, self-evidently, retirement is also a risk factor for those living alone who have previously been engaged in regular work. Single people – compared to those who live with someone – are 1.6 times more likely to be lonely if they live alone, and 5.2 times more likely to be lonely if they are widowed. (Age UK, 2018). Keeping in touch with ex-colleagues is not an entirely satisfactory strategy as such relationships are limited by the fact that there is no longer a commonality of work. Finding a new community in which to be comfortable may be challenging without the familiar structure and routine imposed by work.

Saying 'goodbye' to work

Many workplaces organize a retirement event for anyone leaving, and sometimes offer a gift. This is a kind of ritual, with the intention of showing gratitude for what has been given, and the receiver of such a gift may hopefully feel this is a mark of appreciation. Many transitions have rituals – the birth of a baby is marked in many cultures, weddings are celebrated, and funerals, whether religious or secular, mark out the value of a life and offer the mourners a way of saying goodbye. So, among other things, a ritual marks a transition from 'what was' to a new order of things. CAT therapy pays particular attention to endings. The client is helped to anticipate that the therapeutic relationship and all the work that has been done together will finally end. One of the things that helps this transition is the practice of offering a goodbye letter – sometimes an exchange of letters – that summarizes what may have been achieved and points to a future beyond therapy, in which the client can build on the experience of therapy in their own particular way.

The idea of a 'no send' letter (as explained earlier) addressed to your work-life over the years may be a useful exercise. This would be just for your own interest and possible benefit. It doesn't have to be wholly positive – it could include regrets for mistakes or anger for difficult situations. But the idea is to be honest – about what you will miss, what you won't miss, and perhaps what you are looking forward to in a new post-work life. I have included my own letter as an example of what I mean:

> *Dear Working Life,*
>
> *When I think back to the various jobs I have done – research, teaching, psychotherapy, each of you has given me very precious gifts.*
>
> *When I think back to my first job, my heart was not really in you, dear research, so I thank you for your patience. Thanks go also to you, my teaching posts, I am so glad that you taught me how to explain things and engage even a classroom of disaffected students.*
>
> *But my biggest thanks go to you, my psychotherapy career, and what you have offered me. I have had amazing colleagues who have supported me, challenged me and taught me so much. (I also would like to thank the one or two not-so-helpful colleagues who taught me the precious lesson of choosing whether to fight a battle or move on with life.) Similarly, a big thank you to you, my clients over the years – for*

sharing your stories and helping me understand your vulnerabilities. And that in turn has helped me to understand myself a bit more. And thanks to you, dear clinicians, whom I have supervised, who have also stimulated, challenged and sometimes confounded me, though usually we have found a collaborative way forward.

I want to say sorry to you, those clients who I couldn't help – I hope you are alright and have found some solace somewhere. It makes me sad to write this.

So, I will miss you all, the camaraderie of work, the shared vision and the frustrations of working in the NHS. And especially you, my clients over the years.

I am finding it difficult to retire. I have done a bit of part-time work and that helps soften the blow of the finality of retirement. But I have begun to find the beginnings of a new chapter – perhaps the last chapter of my life. There are things I wasn't encouraged to do at school although I enjoyed them – singing and painting are important new ventures. I might write too. I love having time to potter. I might go on a long-distance cycle ride. Or go on a safari. It's nice to feel open to these projects.

I am a very (happily) active grandma but this needs watching as I will do what I always do – take on too much and forget that time may be running out for me.

My love and good wishes to all who have been part of my working life,

Henrietta

Going forwards: what helps?

As discussed, it is not the case that all retirees experience a loss of identity. Plenty welcome the freedom to develop earlier talents or take up interests abandoned because paid work took priority. Others are pleased for reasons of finance, and interested to reduce formal work to a few days a week or take up self-employed work similar to their employed status. But even if retirement is staggered there comes a time when workers decide – or are forced – to 'hang up their boots' and think again. How can those of us who are retiring move on?

1. A psychological reckoning

Humans like continuity – it is predictable and, to that extent, safe. Letting go of work needs to be accommodated. It may be, like the example of the fireman above, that the loss of work feels unsettling. If work is an attachment, then the loss of this attachment needs to be mourned. This is not to suggest that individuals just feel grief, rather, as already discussed, there may be a mix of emotions including relief and excitement. Alexander Schulman, former editor of *Vogue*, stated: 'It's odd to be a former something' (Segalov, 2022). A psychological reckoning is a way of taking stock of a former life in preparation for what comes next. The importance of respect and compassion for one's true feelings needs to be recognized. As in all transitions, earlier life events may be evoked and may need to be processed. Are there regrets, lost opportunities, or envy of others or of a younger generation? All these things need to be processed.

The psychological needs to go alongside a physical reckoning. Those of us who are retiring are likely to be older, the body is therefore less strong and statistically more vulnerable. Post-work life needs to be planned in the context of physical capabilities, and if living with a partner, their health also needs to be taken into consideration.

2. Know yourself

So many people say after retirement that they are so busy that they have no idea how they fitted work into their lives at all. Usually, this is said with a sense of wonder and achievement but it may be worth reflecting on a particular personality style and whether a person is unwittingly repeating a role or a procedure that was – and is – uncomfortable or unproductive. For example, the person who felt burdened and stressed out by taking on a lot of responsibilities at work may well find that this tendency continues beyond the bounds of work. Or it may be that the person who is unfulfilled at work finds that a post-work life is also unfulfilling. Taking the first example, Figure 5.5 illustrates a reciprocal role state of mind which could drive these patterns, together with perpetuating behaviours. Strategies ('exit' procedures) are suggested in order to find new and better ways forward.

Figure 5.5: An overwork procedure

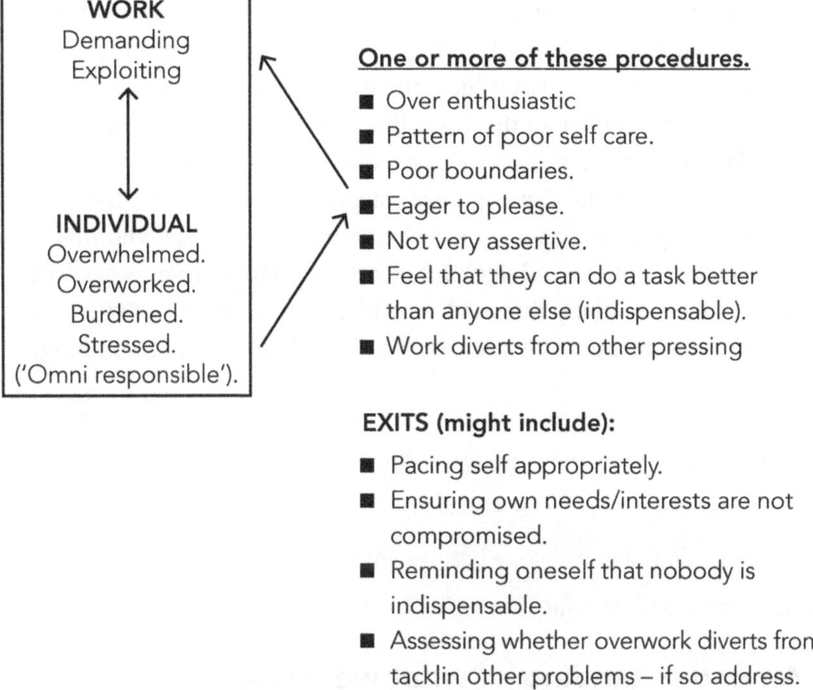

3. Education: be prepared

Much of the research on retirement stresses the need for preparation for this life transition with corresponding better adjustment and higher self-esteem post-retirement (Reitzes, 2004; Wang, 2014). The Calouste Gulbenkian Foundation (2019) recognizes that retirement has a significant impact on people's lives and well-being. They have offered courses in the middle years of employment as a way of helping employees stay in work longer but also plan for retirement by thinking about future needs. Both courses produced good results for future retirees and had unexpected benefits for employers too. The gains included better kindness to self, improved well-being, increased positivity in attitudes to retirement, realistic goals, and more talking to friends and family. Interestingly, there were gains for employers too – employees were very positive about this support and reported better (pre-retirement) 'work-life balance' which prevented burnout and meant they operated better while still at work.

While money isn't everything, enough money to enjoy the retirement you plan is clearly important. One survey showed that 61% of Britons under sixty-six have no idea what their pension will be and most overestimate their retirement income (Wagstyl, 2022). So, preparation for retirement does include working out what income you will have in order to do the things you would like to do. Unfortunately, final salary pensions are now largely a thing of the past and individuals are responsible for their own 'pension pots'. Cernik (2022) suggests that there is a taboo about discussing money as it evokes shame in many people who then subsequently do not seek advice. But clearly, money represents security and while there are many things to do which cost nothing, activities like travel (often on the bucket list of retirees) need financial underpinning.

Exercise

1. You have all the money you want – how do you spend it?
2. You have ten years to live – how will this change your life?
3. You have 24 hours to live, what are your regrets?

(Taken from *The Financial Times* (2019) attributed to George Kinder.)

4. An understanding of what we value

Exploring our values, including those we hold about work, relationships and leisure, can offer an important way to help manage this time of transition. Personal values are the things that are most important to us. They provide us with direction about how we want to live our lives. They play a role in shaping our goals, priorities and identity. Values are influenced by your own beliefs, as well as by your family, friends and society. Some of these values may have been expressed in the job that we have done; others we may hold dear because of the person we are and the experiences we have had. If such values are identified as important, then how can these be transferred into our post-work lives? A number of therapies promote the idea that human beings need to accept and understand what has happened in the past and identify how they feel about these experiences, but then move on to thinking about a future based on the values they hold. So, the suggestion is, while we may search around for something to do in retirement, that something will be more fulfilling and productive if it is in line with our values. The exercise below has some suggestions about how to identify new activities in line with personal values.

Exercise

Identify your values in relation to each of the following:

- Work (for example, I valued having a sense of achievement, and I valued my colleagues).
- Relationships (for example, I value trust, friendship, time with the family, personal space and community activities).
- Your personal growth or learning (I value active learning and reading).
- Leisure or interests (for example, I value freedom, being challenged, being creative etc).

Write down your answers and then choose three or four. How could these values be expressed in post-work activities?

Get-a-life Tree (Zelenski, 2022)

The get-a-life tree suggests drawing a 'tree' of activities that were once valued and are now perhaps discontinued. There may be limitations of age or health that preclude reengagement with such activities after retirement, but its goal is to find similar activities that could be taken up and enjoyed. Are these activities in line with your value base as described in a previous exercise?

Exercise

Using the prompt questions, you may like to draw your own get-a-life tree.

Figure 5.6 (after Zelenski, 2022)

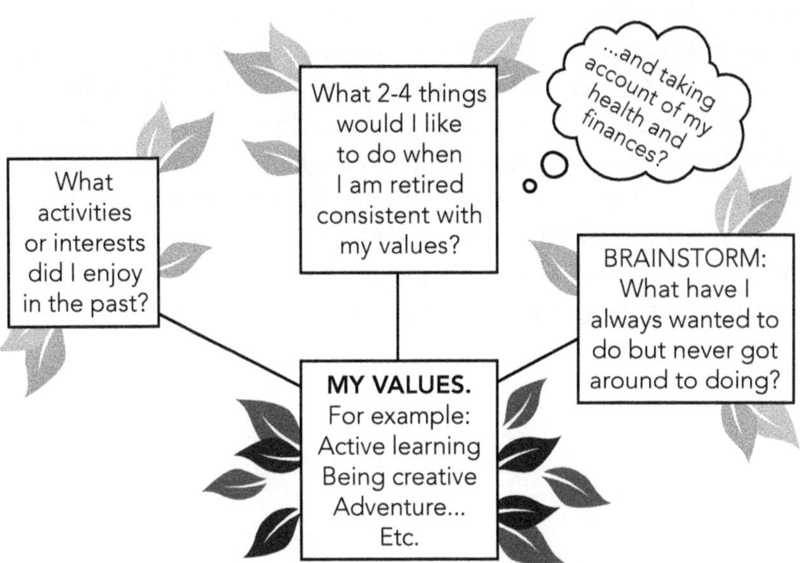

What happens if a retirement project doesn't go to plan?

The decision regarding what is wanted from free time in retirement is one thing, but there may be factors preventing these plans from coming to fruition. So, while some people return to full or part-time employment, or set up in business on their own, to improve their sense of well-being, others have no choice. Similarly, many in their late sixties have care responsibilities for elderly parents or for grandchildren or for a partner who has health difficulties and who needs significant support, which we will discuss further in Chapter 7. There are of course rewards for being needed by family members. However, it may be important to carve out time for oneself in these circumstances in practical ways so that a post-work phase of life contains some time for personal pleasures or ambitions too. An understanding of the potential risk of prioritizing care for others and compromising one's own needs may be enough to set some personal limits

Case study: Jackie

Jackie grew up in a loving family but her needs were overshadowed by a younger brother with special needs. Sadly, he died when he was in his early twenties. Jackie and her husband ran a small hotel and, on retirement, sold the business for a profit. Jackie's learned behavioural patterns (procedures) were to put others before herself without complaint, but this 'bottling up' of feelings and subjugation of her own needs ('put the customers first') led to many episodes of depression throughout her adult life. She and her husband planned to buy a camper and travel in their retirement but he developed vascular dementia and these plans were put on hold. Jackie put on a brave face but developed another debilitating depression. Rather than prescribe antidepressants again, Jackie's GP referred her to the local clinic and she was offered CAT therapy. Through this therapy, Jackie could see that she was about to do what she had always done – looking after others (her husband, specifically) at the expense of her own wishes Figure 5.7.

Figure 5.7: Jackie's map

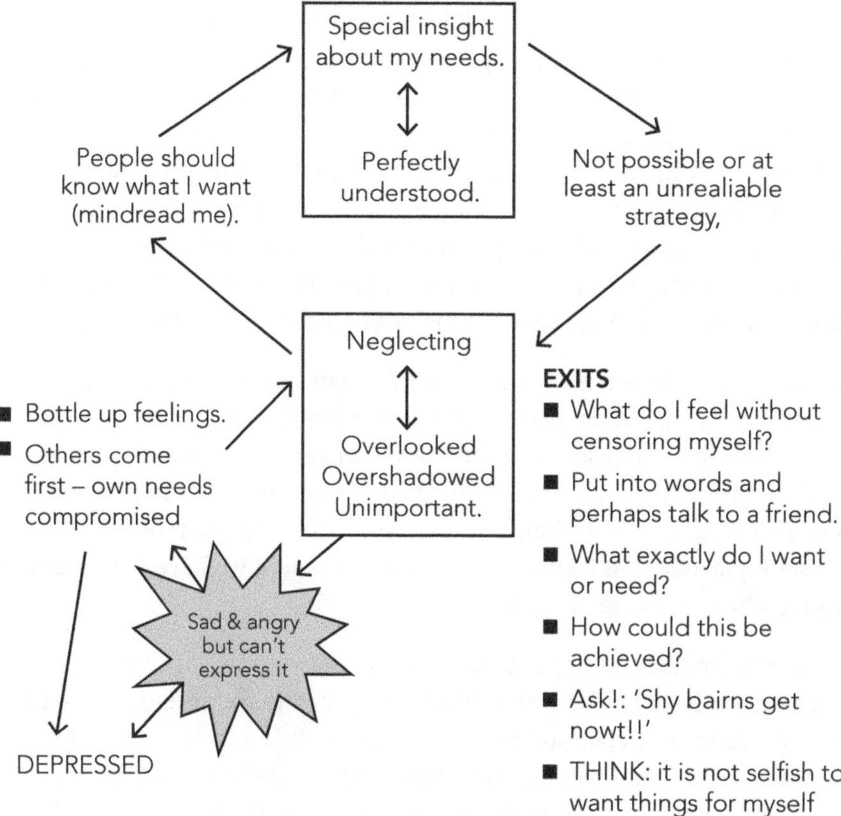

With some hesitation, Jackie began to talk about how cheated she felt that her retirement was being spoiled by her husband's health difficulties and how she was angry with him for getting ill, although she realized that it was not his fault. The therapist wondered about whether she had to give up her goal of travelling and whether this could be achieved without buying a campervan. Jackie thought that she and her husband could enjoy day trips together if they just invested in a larger car and she also thought she might dare to ask a cousin if he would stay for a few days with her husband while she planned a city break. So, while this was not the dream retirement they had planned, it was a good compromise and Jackie's mental health improved as she realized that she could be an active agent in planning her future whatever the difficulties.

Summary

This chapter is about a phase of a life characterized by 'letting go'. It may be that this is a complete letting go or a staggered withdrawal. Given most of us – in contrast to previous generations – have reasonable expectations of longevity and good health, there is more to come. Some people greet retirement with high expectations and can at last find time to do what they have always wanted to do. But this suggests that there has been a plan in mind for some time, even if it was not a formal one. And for those who stagger retirement, which 'sugars the pill', there will come a moment when they have to relinquish what they have done for many years.

CAT helps us make sense of our relationship with work and its meaning in our lives. For many of us, work will have been central to our identity for much of our lives, and served a central role in supporting our self-esteem. As with other step-changes in life, the loss of work may confront us with behavioural patterns that limit or restrict our lives – for example, the overwork procedure in Figure 5.5, or a pattern where we have got used to putting others first (Figure 5.7).

Retirement provides an opportunity to discover new ways of coping and enriching our lives for the better. I have suggested that this letting go – or loss – needs to be accommodated and accepted. It is a mourning, since this stage of life is not coming back. Grasping the reality of this is easier for some than others, as is accepting the range of emotions engendered (sadness, anger, disappointment, envy and anxiety, as well as more positive ones – gratitude, relief, excitement, perhaps?) that accompany this letting go. How we have coped with other life-stage transitions may have a bearing on how this particular transition can be managed.

Above all, it is a change in role, and this is a question that often engages people. It can stick in the gullet to say: 'Well I used to be…'. But this confusion regarding 'who am I now' is also a rich seam to explore. Perhaps it is helpful to explore it tangentially. What are your values? For example, as I have been writing this I realize I need some adventure in my life, that I would be lost if I didn't have a project that meant I was actively learning. Whatever I do next needs to encompass these values. For others, peacefulness, creativity, or exploring new worlds might be important. Sometimes it is helpful to go back to one's adolescence – a life stage when identity begins to crystalize – and consider what talent was discarded because of the need to take up a job to earn money. There is now an opportunity to pick up and develop these 'dropped stitches'.

Preparation is key, including practical preparation such as how much income you have and how this will affect future projects. Health is important and future plans will obviously be affected by this, which is considered in more detail in Chapter 7. And for couples, it may be as well not to assume that more time together is necessarily better. It is important to talk together about a shared new life.

As I wrote earlier, CAT is a therapy that attends to endings carefully. In a good-enough therapy, an ending is anticipated and planned for. It may be helpful to consider other endings during a life – leaving school, the loss of being a couple as children come into a relationship, bereavements… and consider how these have been managed. Were there things you would do differently with hindsight? Such insights are significant. An honest exploration of feelings, and of the person you are, including your value base, practical considerations, and a ledger of losses and gains, all auger well for the next as-yet unwritten chapter called 'retirement'.

Chapter 6: Once upon a time in Stepney – the legacy of complex trauma

Paul Catlin

Editor's note: *In this chapter, Paul generously shares some of his life story. Despite a legacy of complex, lifelong trauma, Paul found hope, meaning, and new possibilities in later life through having CAT with Ellen, with benefits that continue to unfold. Despite widely held beliefs that at his age he was 'past it' and it was too late to change, Paul's story shows how growth and change are possible, despite age or complexity of earlier painful life events. Paul's chapter offers a first-person narrative account, reflecting the early sessions of CAT, which allowed space for in-depth exploration of life experiences to aid with processing, witnessing, and gaining objectivity, all critical to the therapeutic process in later life. In the UK's National Health Service secondary mental health care, we frequently meet people in their later years who have never shared their life experiences. All too often distress in later life and dementia settings is dismissed as age or disease-related rather than linked to early abusive and/or neglectful relational experiences. We will also explore more of this in the next chapter on caring.*

Paul's story also highlights how CAT attends to social and cultural influences which were abusive and damaging, notably prevalent and pervasive for people of his age range - such as the institutionalised brutality across education, health, religious, social care, policing that so many older adults faced, for example, when born out of wedlock, having mixed heritage, and in poverty. CAT attends carefully and explicitly to these different factors, helping to increase compassion and bringing stories of strength and resilience into one's narrative. For clinicians, gaining a more thorough account of people's early relational experiences within the social and cultural contexts they lived is essential when considering the care and treatment that might be needed.

> *'It is easier to build strong children than to repair broken men.'*
>
> Frederick Douglass

A guy walks into a consultation room: the fading late-afternoon light casting a long shadow across the room, a shrouded backdrop – an appropriate tableau reflecting my racing thoughts and inner emotions at the time. 'What would it take to ever rid me of these seemingly insoluble issues forever haunting me? These wretched feelings of existential crisis and imminent forebodings, unwelcome travelling companions throughout life's journey, possessing an unrivalled capacity to affect and disrupt without notice or warning in so many aspects of my life.

Disappointment. Compulsive thoughts in the guise of earnest belief and conviction of any number and manner of calamitous misfortunes lay in waiting. This, I believed and came to accept, was my truth; this accursed poisonous legacy my due inheritance. An intangible hidden presence, my very own Trojan horse hiding in plain sight just waiting patiently for an opportunity to impose itself upon me once again. So, for contextual purposes as to my reasoning for my initial scepticism about therapy, a brief synopsis of my backstory is deemed necessary…

My parents: a mother hailing from London's East End, born the youngest of twelve children from the most humble of backgrounds imaginable. Her life's ambition, sadly unfulfilled, was to work abroad as a Christian missionary. My father hailed from a markedly different background – the scion of a middle-class Nigerian family sent to the UK to study following in the footsteps of his father, my grandfather, with a familial expectancy of returning home after graduating with a first-class degree as a precursor for assuming a senior position in the post-colonial Civil Service. But fate, destiny, kismet, call it what you will, intervened. He happened to meet and fall in love with my mother. However, the prevailing racial climate and attitudes that existed within post-war British society at the time meant that their relationship was tragically doomed to failure.

My teenage mother, now separated from my father, was ostracized and cast out from the family home in shame, ostensibly for renouncing the Roman Catholic faith she was born into. This was as risible and hypocritical a renunciation as one might be as unfortunate to have to confront. Racism. A judgement I formed at an early age, courtesy of various members of my mother's family, to comprehend the depth of the utter ill-feeling and contempt they felt and frequently expressed, about the ethnicity of my distant father. And because of this, my teenaged mother was now left destitute, cast out of her family home alone into a bleak, unforgiving, uncaring world. Alone, that is, except for her two infant offspring; me, aged fifteen months, and a younger sibling - then aged three months - to care for. Forced by cruel circumstance to live a wretched hand-to-mouth existence, as public records have since revealed. Her most urgent daily priority was ensuring overnight shelter for herself and her two children. This, at a time when newsagents windows shamefully featured advertisements for rented accommodation proclaiming, 'No blacks, no dogs, no Irish', as an acceptable moral standard, with, 'No children' as an additional precluding caveat.

It's not too difficult to imagine the humiliating travails my mother, little more than a child herself, was facing. A single mother? ...Shock... Horror!... With two mixed-race babies... Moral disgust!... Born out of wedlock too... More clutching at pearls. Her futile enquiries to rent accommodation inevitably greeted with censorious, callous words of rebuke and reproach. The physical and emotional toll she would have undergone during this traumatic period, I believe, was an indirect cause for her premature demise. At this point, one must also take into account the dearth of welfare provision available to single mothers who had found themselves facing identical straitened circumstances in the post-war interim. Most tellingly, newspaper reportage at the time of my mother's subsequent court appearance (having subsequently been charged with child abandonment) makes crystal clear the disquiet and concern surrounding this matter, as revealed in the closing remarks of the Chief Stipendiary Magistrate at Old Street magistrates court issuing a demand for explanations from the NSPCC, several local authorities, as well as various church mother and baby charities in denying her shelter.

As a consequence, finding herself in the most desperate of situations, she had been obliged to 'go missing', culminating in her abandoning my younger brother while he was in hospital being treated - as the medical records note drily at the time - for 'failure to thrive'. And to compound matters further, with her abject state of mind precipitated by the pitiful circumstances she had now found herself in, she was forced to abandon me. Like my brother, I too was ailing, stricken with pleurisy and a collapsed lung. She had left me in a pram on the landing of a tenement building in Kings Cross and disappeared into the winter night. Some little comfort, but at least offering merciful sanctuary from the seasonal elements in the hope and belief that I would soon be found. My cries of distress led to my eventual discovery by residents, and I was found in my pram in a puddle of faeces and urine. I was rushed immediately to hospital where I was to spend the following three months. Thereafter, as a 'foundling', I was consigned to Ladywell orphanage in South London. Pertinently, decisions made at the time by those responsible for my future welfare incurred significant collateral damage as they led to estrangement from my younger brother. It was not until after launching my own investigation in my late twenties that were we finally reunited.

My brother and I, then virtual strangers to one another, grew up in markedly differing circumstances. Both our parents had tragically predeceased us at an indecently young age. My father, by now relocated to Manchester, succumbed to tuberculosis aged twenty-eight. Our mother died four years earlier in what I passionately believe were unexplained and highly questionable circumstances, at just twenty-one years of age.

And what of me? Aged five, once again fate was to cruelly intervene (confirmed after examination of the heavily redacted Social Services records chronicling my early life and adoption, and released into my possession in the mid-noughties). My maternal grandmother, uncle, and his young wife, for their own questionable motives, belatedly sought custody of me at the same time as another much kinder older couple who had previously collected me from the orphanage to spend weekends at their home in the leafy suburbs on a routine basis, intent on eventually making this arrangement a legally permanent adoption. This outcome was sadly not destined to be. I was taken from the orphanage and transplanted into my maternal family's dysfunctional, surreal, toxic household located in the bomb-scarred dockland landscape of the Isle of Dogs in London's East End – at that time 100% Caucasian. Given that my grandmother, along with my maternal aunts and uncles, had cruelly banished my mother to her eventual fate, the question has to be broached: what was their motive in seeking my adoption?

Their adoption of me would prove to have profound ramifications. The transparent unsuitability of both adoptive parents has since been made clear in my Social Care documents, with a corollary acknowledging my welfare as an adopted child to be a matter of some concern, which served only to put more kindling on the bonfire of insanities my adoption had created. To summarize: physical, emotional, and racist treatment repeatedly suffered while in my foster parent's care, in lockstep with a supporting cast of male authoritarian figures i.e. teachers, police officers. Foremost among my issues was an instinctive distrust and visceral fear and loathing of establishment, institutions and their authority figures. My contrary and reckless behaviour had become customary with a fearless readiness to actively engage in confrontation in opposing all, and any, perceived representatives of an amorphous 'Establishment'. Of course, in the cold light of day, this appears illogically self-destructive. Although my 'acting out' was not strictly in my best interests, untreated over a prolonged period, my self-destructive conduct had become so ingrained within my psyche, and meant that growing up as an angry young man I consequently morphed into an even angrier older man.

The second factor that I personally consider to be a fundamental cause of the subsequent dysfunctional trajectory of my adult life, was that, growing up, I was routinely deprived of so much of what is considered to be crucial for a child to thrive. Love, affection... forget about it! Food and decent clothing – no. In CAT, I came to understand this in terms of a *Depriving-to-Deprived* reciprocal role. The connection between childhood food deprivation and my eating disorder was what brought me to CAT initially. Likewise, forced by obligation to wear ragged clothes and shoes, usually second-hand, for weeks and days at a time, much to the collective derision of my peers, left me with a residual complex about my appearance and how others perceived me. So it's hardly surprising, despite displaying early signs of academic promise, reared as I was in this highly dysfunctional environment, I became an extremely disruptive pupil during my latter years in primary school, resulting in my being sent to boarding school. This consisted of three classes and a restrictive curriculum catering for forty male pupils. Within three years of my entry, I found myself in the top class delegated by my teacher to teaching much older pupils to read.

My ambition, other than typical schoolboy aspirations to be a footballer, was to be a journalist, but this was denied me upon leaving school as GCSE exams were not considered part of the curriculum so I left school without any qualifications to offer prospective employers. Although I had expressed a wish to attend college, this initiative was dismissed by my foster parents making it clear that, if I wished to continue living in the family home, then I would have to go out to work and contribute to the household finances. So the building sites and factories beckoned as

I could not possibly begin to afford a bedsit on my first wage – the 2023 equivalent of £5.50 a week. I must take my fair share of responsibility, too, for my descent into criminal activity.

By the time I reached ten years of age, I was attending weekly sessions with a psychiatrist – for one so young in those more unenlightened times I believe a comparatively unheard of event – while those responsible for my troubled behaviour had somehow managed to evade official investigation or sanction. This might, or not, have been the decisive factor for my being packed off to a boarding school for 'maladjusted boys' – with some members of staff with paedophilic tendencies, others ever willing to inflict corporal punishment upon their young charges for the most minor of transgressions. 'Maladjusted'; to this day this classification of me remains personally unacknowledged and fiercely refuted. However, the stigma that the label confers lingers, and was deeply felt until recently. The primary reason given at the time for consigning me to Heathermount School was 'chronic bed wetting' issues. Hardly surprising when most nights would find me in bed laying awake fearfully listening out for my foster father invariably staggering home from the pub, praying fervently that he wouldn't come into my squalid bedroom after his drink-fuelled rants at my foster mother and grandmother. On occasions, it would conclude with my bedroom door crashing open and without specific reason or explanation culminate in him, a fully-grown male, raining blow after blow upon my head and body all the time screaming racist invective in a drunken fury. Memorably, on one specific occasion, smashing to pieces the few meagre toys I possessed. This left me with the enduring feeling that his incomprehensible hatred directed towards me was the consequence of a belief that my existence was somehow indirectly connected to the early death of his closest and favourite sibling, my mother. What is of significance, though, is the inescapable fact that throughout my near five years at boarding school, I wet the bed on one occasion, just once.

My being sent to boarding school was engineered by my ever-scheming foster mother for her own nefarious motives. The methods of punishment she inflicted upon me were no less destructive upon my nascent psyche and took the form of what is now termed as 'passive aggression'. But denial or restrictions of food were her favoured punishment 'du jour'. This was made worse by the apparent relish she displayed with each mouthful she took before my very uncomprehending eyes. The unstinting episodes of 'silent treatment' were another of her 'go-to' punishments, and also had a particularly tormenting effect upon me. To be met with this wall of silence confused, frustrated and maddened me in equal measure. The recollection of that one occasion when for months she didn't utter a single word to me only to inexplicably break her 'vow of silence' without giving any warning or explanation (apologies out of the question) resuming our mutual verbal interaction as if nothing had ever happened. These abuses, along with so many other torments imposed as a matter of routine and often for no discernible reason, were the wellspring for the nascent sense of incandescent rage emerging from within and much to my detriment in later life. The consequences of these physical acts of violence that I was routinely subjected to at home and boarding school – a reflection of the toxic masculinity that growing into adulthood I too readily embraced, in common with many of my chosen peer group. Before the abuse became routine, I was a generally well-behaved and obedient child, willing to run errands, and clean the home – we lived to my undying shame in utmost squalor – attending to the needs of an aged grandmother.

Discovering CAT

None of these experiences would have ever been remotely possible for me to understand so late in life were if not for the lessons bequeathed by CAT. Sitting here before me, over half a century later, this female CAT therapist, looking no older than the second of my three daughters, distinctly middle-class in comparison to my working-class sensibilities (as was every other therapist that had counselled me in the past) and... yet another white person! After all, as a person of mixed heritage, was it not an undeniable fact that it was those from that particular ethnicity who were responsible for a lifetime of abuses perpetuated against me? At that moment, to my blinkered eyes and skewed thought processes, the very notion of there being no common ground existing between us signified clearly to me the odds for bridging the yawning gap in age, class, and gender between us. But I felt that I really did not deserve any better. I thought this previously unfamiliar therapy didn't have a 'cat in hell's chance' (no pun intended) of achieving a positive outcome for me. At my then age (sixty-five), I had undergone all manner of therapeutic and pharmaceutical options previously, none of which had come even remotely close to offering the resolution I so desperately sought.

I had first attended group therapy at a hospital in South London but soon concluded that this particular therapy was totally unsuitable for my particular needs, finding myself increasingly reluctant to speak amidst a veritable Tower of Babel of different voices with so many other animated participants competing to be heard. From then on, having made little, if any, discernible progress for my mental condition, I was fortunate in securing further treatment on a one-to-one basis. This was all based on Cognitive Behavioural Therapy (CBT). My personal issues with CBT stemmed for the most part from what I considered to be the detached nature of the conventional question/answer paradigm, along with the ruminative period that generally ensued afterwards between therapist and service user. The lack of emotional engagement between practitioner and patient meant I rarely, if ever, formed a working connection with those undertaking my treatment, which, in hindsight, caused me to adopt a more circumspect attitude in my responses. It all felt so rigid, sterile even, which my sensibilities felt unable to engage with.

In CAT, we came a long way from that initial impression – of frustration, weary disappointment and, I confess, mild resentment – my thinking, 'Oh no, who have they stuck me with now?' This misplaced rush to judgement had no basis for validity and was based purely upon my own misperceptions about seemingly white, middle-class professionals and presumed cultural disconnections. I mistakenly believed this would inhibit mutual communication and understanding between us, thereby proving to be a waste of my time and my attempts of making progress with long-existent mental health issues given the relative disparities in our ages, respective backgrounds, life experiences and ethnicity. But what made it possible to overcome my scepticism was the fact that these differences between us were named and explored in the therapy.

Why did CAT help? The sterling work of the therapist who treated me, whose diligence, clinical skill, and combined with that most invaluable of components...empathy. Our first meeting proved to be a real 'sliding doors' moment. I so nearly got up from my chair and walked out of the room expressing my ingrained scepticism about the professional capabilities of the young therapist sitting before me, however, a sense of common courtesy persuaded me otherwise. So, there I stayed, in my seat figuring that I should just have to 'suck it up', after all, was it not my trusting naivety that had placed me here in the first place? But with the assured intention that I certainly wouldn't be returning for a second instalment. But the longer I stayed, and by now obliged to listen as she outlined the methodology and general aims of CAT and what the therapy had to offer in achieving quantifiable outcomes, something happened. Here was someone now speaking calmly to me in a language and assured manner that for the first time in therapy intuitively I could begin to relate to.

With my CAT therapist, I came to understand that my experiences of trauma and abuse left me feeling that I couldn't have what I needed or wanted. Depriving myself of things, including food, was a target problem for the therapy. I learned that when I deprived myself, this fed into my sense that I was inferior and deserved no better, like a self-fulfilling prophecy. From a young age, I created a veneer of being 'tough and egotistical', as a protective armour. However, this meant my feelings and needs were hidden and never attended to, leaving me feeling misunderstood, overlooked and deprived, and feeding into my sense of shame and anger. Integral to our work, and what CAT offered that other therapies had not, was the exploration of the wider social determinants of my troubles. It was the first time my life history and story had been understood in the context of the wider social culture and milieu – generational racism growing up in an all-white environment, toxic masculinity, religion and misogyny that forced my mother to abandon my brother and me, and post-war poverty. These things were explored, not only in relation to my life experiences, but also in relation to the therapeutic relationship between myself and the therapist. I could see how these relational experiences were re-playing in the present day, and in the therapeutic relationship.

CAT helped me to understand and accept accountability for my actions, which were as a consequence of injustices wrought against me in earlier years. Working together, I developed the ability to forgive myself, and to forgive others, and for that alone I am eternally grateful. CAT has been invaluable in overcoming a deep sense of shame. As I write now, it becomes ever-more apparent to me how the evolving benefits of CAT are still apparent many years later. CAT took a more holistic approach with an innovative and interactive approach to communication.

The CAT tools – maps and letters – are, in my opinion, an effective communication medium between therapist and patient. Before treatment I considered myself a 'helpless and forlorn case'. When the therapist asked questions of me while directing my attention to relevant aspects of the map, I felt that my critical thought processes showed a marked improvement as a result of being able to see, as well as hear, bringing a sense of 'joined-up thinking'. The benefits of being able to take the map home between sessions (with additions) and consult and evaluate at leisure meant that I was able to return the following week and contribute more to our sessions together which, in all probability, would not have been the case otherwise. This helped to maintain the ongoing narrative in between weekly sessions. There was a warmth in the overall approach compared to the studied impassiveness that I had encountered before. But most important was the nature and quality of our mutual discourse with each other. This, when compared with other therapies, allowed me to speak freely about my life – for which the therapist exhibited Olympian levels of patience – and was in retrospect of massive benefit to me in allowing me to explore multiple aspects of my life in depth. It allowed me to ask questions too, which, in marked contrast with previous experiences, just felt more inclusive. Of course, this did not miraculously occur overnight, but in time my trust in her abilities and the process grew exponentially.

Figure 6.1: Paul's map

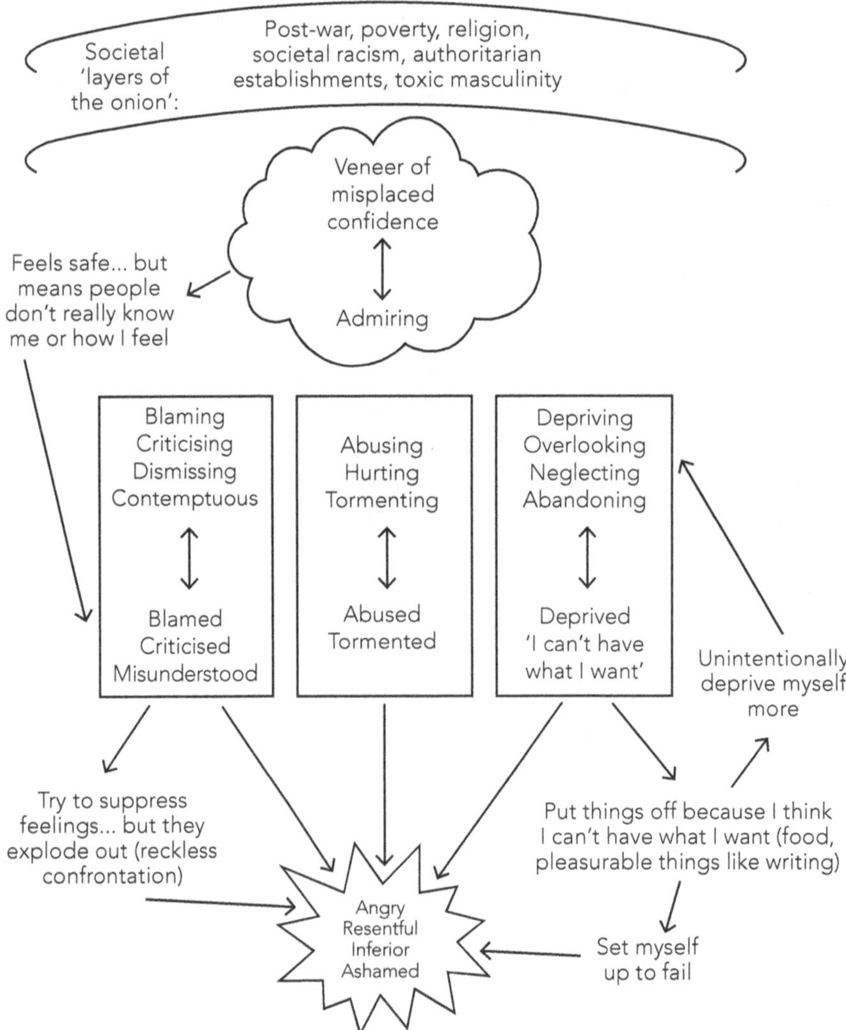

Despite an admittedly limited knowledge of mental health symptoms and counselling, my immediate perception of CAT was that it was holistic. No other form of therapy had remotely succeeded in gaining this unalloyed confidence, but I like to think she saw something in me that few had done before, going all the way back to my schooldays and teachers, and most others going forward. The attention and skills dedicated on my behalf with the critical insights acquired during our time together is duly acknowledged for the therapist's role in enabling me to begin to heal the open wounds of a broken soul as I traverse the unknown terrain of life at a later age. This is a rare gift of incalculable, lasting value bestowed upon me. The letter the therapist wrote to me as my treatment neared its end is one that I will always treasure as a keepsake. Even now as I re-read it, it evokes bitter-sweet feelings within. However, this is no bad thing. The words contained within explain to me how far I have come and where I once was. And just as profoundly state: 'We are all a work in progress'. Age is no barrier to changing for the better and finding a new sense of purpose and role in life.

So now, as the consequence of life experience, I might always be considered a 'work in progress', and without claiming CAT to be a 'one-size-fits-all' panacea. But, when taking into account the substantive consequential effect upon someone of my background and life history, one hopes that those reading this might award Cognitive Analytical Theory the most serious consideration. Because from my own experience, I can authoritatively state, as principal beneficiary, my eternal gratitude that for once, just this once, spurning habitual impulses, I chose to remain seated in my chair rather than walking out of the room on that gloomy autumn day.

Before I started CAT, I had started writing my memoir, to make sense of my life and history. Writing stories has always made me feel safe and secure. As a child, I spent an unnatural amount of time in tormented solitude, invariably locked away in the squalor of my bedroom. My only means of escape was the safe harbour of my imagination. As I wrote, a world of fantastical possibilities would emerge, transporting me far, far away to another place that was mine, and mine alone. Writing is a lifetime passion of mine, and I continue to write my memoir alongside other writing projects. The peaceful haven of writing has not deserted me. And for that I am grateful, a testament to triumph over adversity, hope and resolution. This is my raison d'etre.

Paul's memoir is named *Disputed Child of an Uncertain Future* in reference to a chapter from *City of Spades* by Colin MacInnes, a book from his London Trilogy depicting life for Nigerian immigrants in London in the 1950s. Paul and his father feature in this book under pseudonyms.

Chapter 7: When health changes – caring and being cared for

Ellen Khan and Michelle Hamill

> '*Caring can be learned by all human beings, can be worked into the design of every life, meeting an individual need as well as a pervasive need in society.*'
>
> Mary Catherine Bateson (daughter of Margaret Mead)

As we have described throughout the book, later life can be a time when coping strategies are challenged by losses and transitions that resonate with earlier experiences of vulnerability and dependency. Paul's chapter offers a deeply personal account of this. In this chapter, we will return to our clinical and professional experiences to explore how CAT sensitively attends to relationship changes that can arise when caring is required in one's later years. When aging brings health changes that increase dependency on another person, relationships can understandably change in all sorts of ways. We have witnessed the most powerful examples of love and deep commitment in our work settings when care needs arise, alongside the struggles and despair that such changes can bring.

Challenges can arise for both the person who needs increasing levels of 'care', and for the person who 'provides the care', where there were previous levels of general independence. For this chapter, we will be focusing on relationships where the need for care by one person in a relationship arises in later life, rather than attending to lifelong caring relationships, as aging in those contexts can bring up other challenges and dilemmas. If you are reading this as someone who cares for a partner or relative in their later years, or are reading as someone who requires others to help you due to a health condition or change of circumstances, then we hope you find some insights into the changing nature of these relationships in this chapter.

Understandably, there is huge variability in how people respond to such relationship changes when the need for care arises. Love can change, and it comes in many different shapes and forms. Some people surprise themselves and rise to the task, adjusting both emotionally and practically as needs change and increase. For others, these changes in dynamic can be overwhelming and result in despair, anger and avoidance – a sense that 'this isn't what I signed up for!' Resentment and resignation can arise, resulting in depression and at times neglect of the person in need of care. All relationships naturally have their ups and downs, where feelings of disconnection come and go. However, where there are longstanding issues in relationships – for example, where things have been fraught, neglectful, or abusive – the ability to provide or receive care requires particular care and thinking, including determining whether a caring relationship is even possible.

As psychologists in the NHS, we often work with people who have had complicated relationships throughout life, including with the person they are now 'expected' to care for. We use the word 'expected' in this way, as the expectation to care for another is informed and driven by all sorts of relationship and sociocultural factors (e.g. 'blood is thicker than water', 'what would other people say?' and 'till death do us part'), which CAT can hold in mind, while offering some ideas for change to support better well-being, for both parties. When relationships have been strained or complicated, the ability to care with dignity and compassion may feel impossible, not least when feeling bound by a sense of duty.

For example, perhaps you are an adult child who did not experience your parents or caregivers as emotionally available, or perhaps you experienced them as critical and withholding, and now, because of their changing health, they need care. Or perhaps you are a spouse or partner where control (or lack of control) has been a key feature in your relationship. Such relationship dynamics can result in powerful feelings when the need for care arises in later life, e.g. a tension between feeling obliged to care for the person who you haven't felt cared for you, for whatever reason. It is up to everyone to honestly ask themselves, 'Can I provide care for my relative, despite our history, especially when things have been complicated?' There is no shame in coming to the answer that you cannot provide safe and dignified care to a parent who was neglectful or to a partner who has been controlling. Rather, the best thing you may do in these circumstances is decide that, in your interests and theirs, care by another person or from a formal paid carer is required. Seeking professional help or guidance in such circumstances, if possible, may be helpful.

Figure 7.1 illustrates a carer who had experienced their partner as critical and often withheld attention and affection. When their partner developed a serious health condition and required high levels of care, the expectation to then care for them resulted in feelings of resentment. These feelings led to guilt, which was managed by trying to bury them but, with the pressures of caring, they would fester and brew until they exploded. The carer then became critical and withholding of care towards their partner, which had a detrimental impact on their care needs being met. Guilt would arise again, and the pattern continued. For this carer, the way of managing was to explore the legacy of their relationship experiences, and compassionately validate their feelings. Through these understandings, the decision was made against continuing with caring, instead opting for paid carers and subsequently residential care, which protected the well-being of both people.

Figure 7.1: An example of when caring is not possible

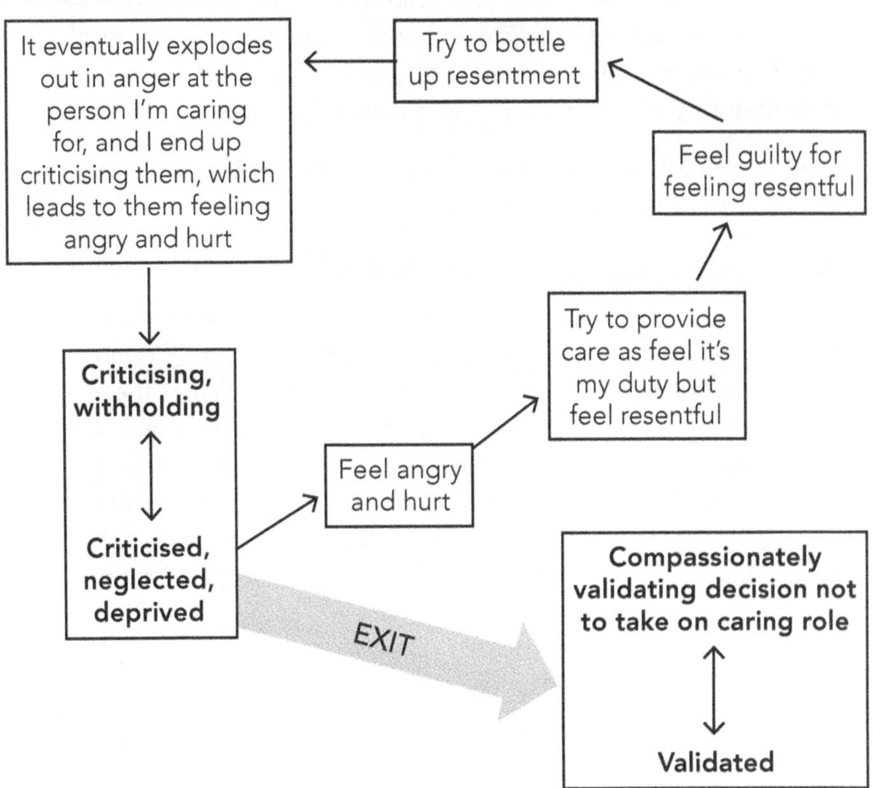

In the next section, we will focus on relationships in which the decision to continue to care has been made and there is a commitment to find a way to manage relationship changes, including challenges, in a way that attends to the well-being and natural limitations of both parties. In terms of the relationships between 'carer' and 'cared-for', we have found that CAT can help to provide a framework to make sense of relationship patterns in the context of both parties' lives. This helps to reduce the risk of re-enactment of limiting or harmful relational patterns – within and between the carer, the person who requires care, and the wider society. New possibilities within the caring role can be explored and developed, and, through its sensitivity to endings, CAT acknowledges and facilitates the associated grieving process, at the end of life, and when conditions are degenerative or terminal. These ideas will be further explored in Chapter 8.

Who cares?

> *'A carer is considered to be anyone who spends time looking after or helping a friend, family member or neighbour who, because of their health and care needs, would find it difficult to cope without this help regardless of age or whether they identify as a carer.'*
>
> Carers Action Plan 2018 – 2020 Supporting carers today, Department of Health and Social Care

How does caring impact on carers?

Unpaid carers provide billions of pounds worth of care across the world. Unpaid informal care provided by friends and family is essential to society and the economy. In a survey of 750 carers across the world, 87% reported finding caring rewarding (Merck, 2021). This may vary across cultural groups. For example, in Islam, older people have a high status, and looking after an older relative is considered a part of religious practice drawing on the principles of cooperation, compassion and mutual support, thereby bringing meaning and a higher sense of purpose (MacKinlay, 2010).

Exercise

What aspects of caring do you find rewarding? What helps you to feel valued and appreciated as a carer?

....

....

....

....

While many carers report satisfaction and a strong sense of purpose within their caring role, caring can also take its toll financially, emotionally, socially and physically. Eight in ten carers said they had felt lonely or socially isolated. Sixty-one per cent said they had suffered ill-health because of caring. In the Carers Worldwide Impact Report (2020), 79% of carers reported anxiety or depression, 48% had neglected seeking support about their health due to a lack of time or money, and 92% worried about money.

Around the world, carers are diverse, meaning that each carer faces a unique set of challenges. As the population gets older, an increasing number of workers and people who are parents themselves (the so-called 'sandwich generation') are providing care during their working life for family members, while also raising children. In the Global Carer Well-being Index study (Merck, 2021) that studied survey responses of seven hundred and fifty carers across twelve countries, 69% of carers in Taiwan were caring for parents, as opposed to other family members. This was significantly higher than the average in the other twelve countries (48% caring for parents) and is thought to be due to Taiwan's super-aged society. This could be taken as a sign of things to come as life expectancy increases across the globe, and both 'carer' *and* 'cared-for' are likely to be older.

The number of carers over the age of sixty-five is increasing more rapidly than the general carer population. Recent polling suggests that there could now be over two million people aged sixty-five or older who are carers in the UK. Older carers – those aged eighty-five and over – are most likely to be carer for someone with dementia (53.6%). Not only does this mean that often both 'carer' and 'cared-for' are older people themselves, each facing the complexities and challenges that later life can bring, but over 50% of carers aged eighty-five and over are also supporting care needs related to physical disabilities, and it is therefore likely that the cared-for person has multiple needs. Carers themselves are also often contending with their own health challenges; in a survey by Carers UK (2019), 60% of carers reported having their long-term health condition or disability compared to 50% of non-carers.

Across the world, women outnumber men when it comes to caring. According to Carers Worldwide (2020), women and girls make up 84% of carers globally. Carers from a black, Asian or minority ethnic group in the UK were more likely to report financial struggles during the pandemic. Carers who identified as LGBTQ+ were more likely to report feelings of loneliness (Carers Worldwide, 2020). This research points to how becoming a carer intersects with other aspects of identity, such as gender, age, disability, ethnicity, sexuality and socioeconomic status, sometimes compounding the challenging parts of caring. In a CAT sense, previous experiences of disadvantage or prejudice may have contributed to harmful relationship roles, including how a person experiences care. Faced with the changing nature of the relationship with the cared-for person, the unpredictability of complex health conditions, and the juggling of daily tasks, carers' well-being can be significantly impacted. Alongside this, carers of older people are contending with the changing nature of the relationship, which may result in feelings of loss.

Exercise

Do you think any aspects of your identity and life experience impact on your experience of being a carer: age (and ageism), ethnicity, gender, religion, (dis)ability, class, sexuality, or financial resources?

....

....

....

....

Being cared for

While a lot has been written about the experience of caring, comparably little has been written about the experience of declining health from a previous level of independence, necessitating the need to be cared for in one's later years. The older people we have worked with have told us of the negative impact of decreasing independence on their mental health, especially when their declining health has stopped them from seeing friends and family, or from doing things they previously enjoyed or from which they have gained a sense of satisfaction. Declining health and increasing reliance on others can also bring about difficult feelings of a loss of control. For some, this compounds a sense of a lack of control in their relationship with the person who is 'caring' for them. This can be particularly challenging when faced with a degenerative condition, such as dementia, in which neither carer nor cared-for have any control over the progression of the illness, and in which the end of the caring relationship usually entails the death of the cared-for person. For people who have previously placed value on being self-reliant, requiring care and support from others in later life can be extremely challenging.

Ivor's story

Ivor, a ninety-two-year-old Jewish man who grew up in London, was referred to therapy by a psychiatrist after he had expressed suicidal thoughts to his GP. In the last eighteen months, Ivor's health had declined rapidly – he had been hospitalised with a heart attack and recently developed rheumatoid arthritis. He was also undergoing investigations for cancer. His mobility had rapidly declined, and he now required a walking frame to mobilise. Until the recent decline in his health, Ivor had been self-sufficient and very active; he had worked until his late seventies, after which he had enjoyed a rich cultural life of theatre trips, art exhibitions and dinners with friends.

Ivor had grown up in what he referred to as a 'high-achieving' family of doctors or lawyers, and he had always been expected to enter one of these professions. He described his parents as 'Victorian', and of the 'stiff-upper-lip generation'. His parents paid for him to attend a private school, which Ivor described as strict and bullying, and there was some anti-Semitism. The teachers used physical punishment and Ivor would be caned for writing with his left hand. The school placed great emphasis on being good at science and maths, but Ivor felt out of place, preferring the arts. He felt inadequate, unhappy and under pressure to achieve, but felt unable to tell his parents that he was not happy at the school as he knew they had stretched themselves financially to pay for it. After leaving school, Ivor went to Cambridge University and subsequently became a solicitor. Ivor married but never had children. He described his marriage as a happy one but said that he and his wife lived rather independent lives and never spoke much about feelings.

Ivor described hating that he was struggling to do things that he used to do easily. He resisted others' attempts to help him, assuming that they 'pitied him'. Ivor's fierce independence and determination to do things in the way he always had, meant that he often ended up not doing them at all, as he found them too difficult to do without help. For example, Ivor struggled to travel on his own to the theatre and sit in his favourite seat, which required him to climb up several steps, so he stopped going to the theatre altogether. He also stopped meeting his friends as he struggled to travel to their favourite restaurant meeting place. This all took its toll on Ivor's mood, and he started to feel that life had no meaning, leading to depression and suicidal thoughts.

In therapy, Ivor initially struggled to talk about how he felt, often resorting to acerbic wit when discussing his current situation. Ivor saw his response to his declining independence as entirely 'to be expected', as if everyone whose health declined would contemplate suicide. However, as we started to unpick things in therapy, he came to understand how, from his early life, he had internalised a demanding way of speaking to himself, pushing himself to achieve, and otherwise criticising and berating himself for being inadequate, just like the little boy at school who was bullied and punished. Ivor came to see that his self-esteem and sense of himself as a good-enough person throughout his life had been founded on being intelligent and high achieving; this made absolute sense as a way of deriving self-esteem in the context of a high-achieving family that valued career success, and a school life of bullying and punishment.

Ivor also realized that he had been 'too busy to think or feel' for much of his life. Being high achieving and busy had worked well for him previously, but now that his health and independence were declining and he was no longer able to function in that way, it unmasked intolerable feelings of vulnerability and inadequacy, to which the only solution for Ivor seemed to be suicide. It made sense that Ivor struggled to articulate and compassionately respond to these difficult feelings, given that his earliest experience of emotions was that of the Victorian 'stiff upper lip'. Ivor had internalized an 'emotionally overlooking' to 'emotionally overlooked' relational role, in which feelings were brushed under the carpet, buried, and not talked about. This left Ivor, and many others of his generation, struggling to acknowledge, talk about or attend to painful feelings and to seek better ways to manage.

Over time in therapy, Ivor was able to develop exits from these unhelpful and restrictive relational patterns, including acknowledging and taking a compassionate stance to the feelings of inadequacy and vulnerability, noticing when he was criticizing and bullying himself and generating more compassionate, validating ways things to say to himself instead, for example, by asking himself what a friend would say to him, or what he would say to a friend in a similar situation. Through attending to those feelings, alongside feelings of grief and loss for the things he now struggled to do, Ivor grew more accepting of the limitations posed by his health. Ivor recognized that he could still connect with the things he valued and enjoyed, albeit in a different way. Whereas before, Ivor had so fiercely resisted help from others, doggedly tried to do things independently in the way he had always done, now he uncovered an interesting paradox – that when he was more accommodating of his needs and his dependence on others, he was able to connect more with the things he'd always enjoyed. For example, Ivor started to invite friends to see him at home instead of meeting them in a restaurant, he realized he could still enjoy going to the theatre if he accepted some help from his wife or friends to get there, and if he sat in a seat near the front reserved for people with mobility problems or disabilities. His depression lifted and he no longer felt suicidal. Ivor felt a sense of achievement in having made changes in his relational responses to changing health and seeking help. Life became meaningful again.

Figure 7.2: Ivor's map

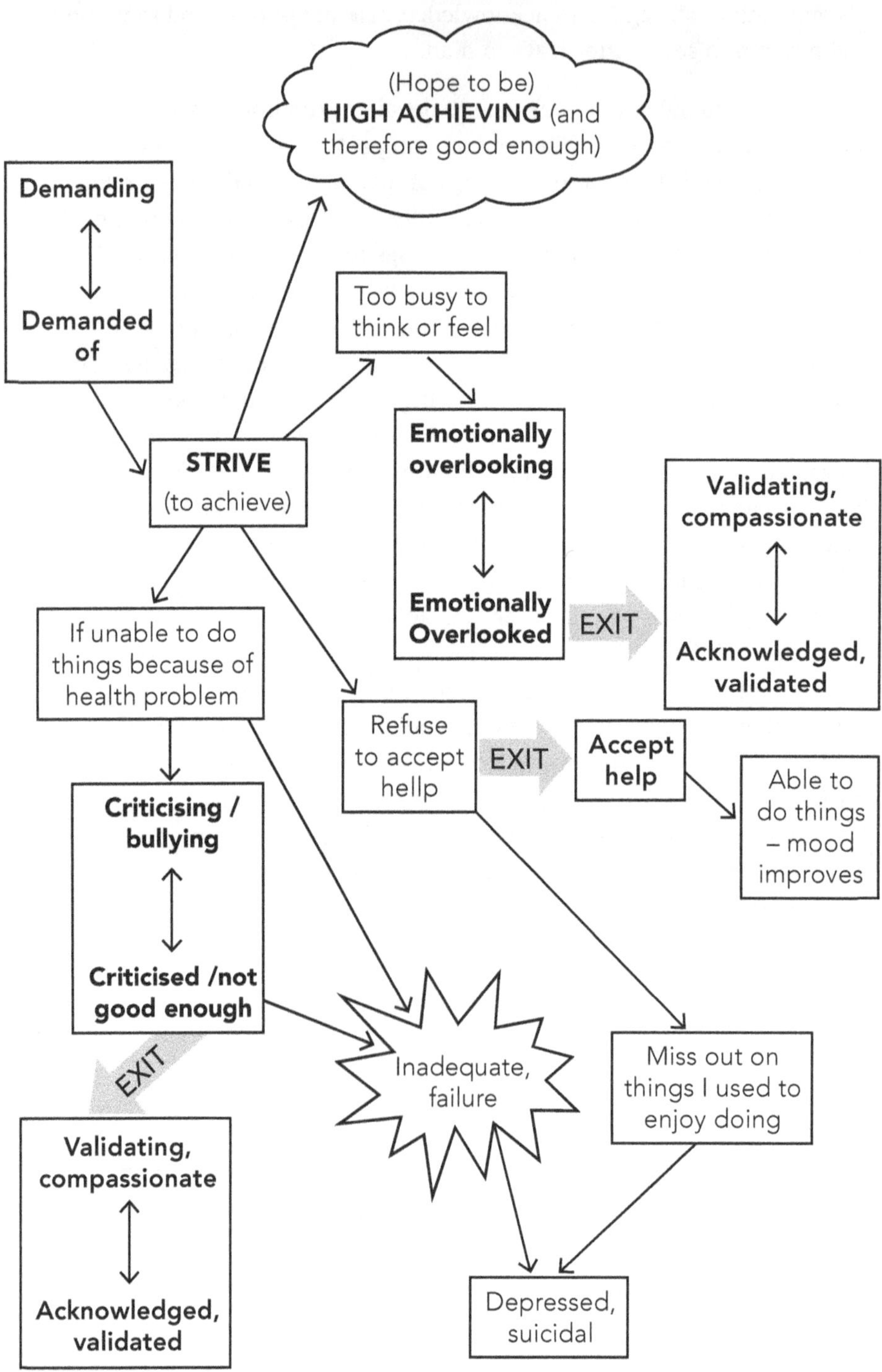

Early trauma and later-life risks

When it comes to older adults who require care, childhood abuse is a risk factor for abuse and neglect by caregivers (Fulmer *et al*, 2005). This requires particular attention in dementia care and highlights the need for sensitivity to signs of early trauma in both the person with dementia and their carers, as well as carer burnout and stress. Supporting caregivers therapeutically can help to mitigate some of these risks and optimize the quality of life for both the person in need of care and the person providing it. Nevertheless, the effects of early trauma and neglect are often missed in later life and misdiagnosed as dementia, depression, personality disorder, somatization and mania (Allers *et al*, 1992; Martinez-Clavera *et al*, 2017). Some carers are shocked to only learn of the trauma history of the person they are caring for in later life, in the context of becoming their carer, when difficulties can come to the fore due to increasing dependence and vulnerability. It is common for experiences of childhood sexual abuse to be disclosed for the first time in later life, after a diagnosis of dementia, or when the person starts to show signs of being re-traumatized during intimate personal care tasks. Early experiences of prejudice and racism can also be triggered by things like receiving care from care workers.

Some studies have found that people with PTSD (post-traumatic stress disorder) have a significantly higher likelihood of developing dementia than those who do not. Though the reason is unclear, this may have something to do with stress-related changes in the brain and central nervous system (Qureshi *et al*, 2010; Yaffe *et al*, 2010). At the same time, the onset of dementia is a risk factor in developing 'delayed-onset PTSD', which refers to the emergence of PTSD, sometimes years after traumatic events occurred (Johnston, 2000; Mittal *et al*, 2001; van Achterberg *et al*, 2001). This delayed onset may be in response to stressors common in later life, from losses including health crises. Combat veterans may be particularly susceptible to late-onset PTSD as they grow older (Davison *et al*, 2016; Davison *et al*, 2006; Ruzich *et al*, 2005). Behavioural disturbances in dementia may be solely put down to disease-related symptoms when the person may be experiencing symptoms of PTSD (Amano & Toichi, 2014; Martinez-Clavera *et al*, 2017).

Having knowledge and a sensitive awareness of a person's history, especially trauma history, is essential to ensure access to appropriate treatments and managing vulnerability while putting safeguards in place concerning risk. It is also helpful in predicting which tasks of caring, for the cared-for person may struggle with most. If a person has had experiences of abuse, oppression or prejudice in their early life, they may be more alert and even hyper-vigilant to these sorts of experiences when receiving care. Understanding this can help to provide more trauma-informed and person-centred care interventions.

Working with carers of people with dementia

Dementia is a progressive neurodegenerative condition resulting in changes in cognition and emotional regulation which interfere with a person's ability to function in everyday life. It is one of the major causes of disability and dependency among older people worldwide. The World Health Organization (2020) estimates that over fifty million people worldwide are living with dementia. As dementia progresses, increasing levels of care are required to support them. Research shows that carers of people with dementia experience more anxiety and depressive symptoms than other carers (Connors *et al*, 2020). The well-being of carers is an important issue for public healthcare, not only because of their central role in the care of people with dementia but also because of the negative health consequences that they may experience as a result of caring. Despite burnout, carers often delay asking for help and neglect their own health needs (Dening, 2012).

Research indicates that the well-being and maintenance of a person with dementia in the community has more to do with the well-being and attitudes of family carers than factors such as the severity of the disease (Clare & Shakespeare, 2004), highlighting the importance of attending to the relational world of the person with dementia and their carer. This becomes even more important when considering the legacy of early trauma and the risk of abuse, as outlined above. Hamill and Mahony (2011) suggest that CAT is well placed to explore the helpful or unhelpful coping strategies used by carers, and CAT's focus on endings can help to consider issues that may arise in the event an illness is terminal or degenerative, such as dementia.

Common procedures in therapy with carers

CAT is well placed to identify longstanding relational patterns, which were at one time adaptive but have become less helpful in the context of caring. Furthermore, CAT helps identify patterns of relating that were present in the relationship between the carer and cared-for person before the health changes and need for care, but which have been brought to the fore in the context of the caring role, and can result in complex and mixed feelings of resentment, guilt, anger or grief. Acknowledging and naming experiences in an open and non-judgemental manner helps to create a space where thinking and reflection become more possible, facilitating adaptations to the demands of caring. In our work with carers, we see several commonly occurring reciprocal role procedures (RRPs):

Overlooking/neglecting to overlooked and neglected

Some carers may come to the caring role in the context of longstanding patterns of neglect of their own needs - physical, emotional or otherwise - and are sometimes drawn (consciously or unconsciously) to the role of carer for this reason. This can result in carers feeling resentful as their needs are repeatedly overlooked, which can then lead to guilt. Patterns like this often link to a dilemma around carers believing their needs are less important so they must be self-sufficient and not ask for help, but then feeling overwhelmed, alone and burnt out. Behavioural and psychological symptoms of dementia such as psychosis, paranoia, agitation and disturbed sleep are also common, further complicating the level of care a person requires and further feeding into carers' needs and feelings being overlooked.

Controlling to controlled

Carers often report feeling helpless in the face of the progressive nature of dementia. In response, carers may seek to establish control, for example, by declining help from others, or controlling their feelings by 'keeping a lid' on them. The practical care tasks involved in caring for a person with dementia can be extremely physically and emotionally demanding and often leave carers too busy to think or feel. While these procedures may help carers feel more in control in the short term, especially in avoiding the painful feelings of loss and grief, in the longer term they lead to carers becoming burnt out or finding themselves in a dilemma whereby their feelings are bottled up to a point that they then explode out in anger or frustration, at times directed towards those they care for. This can lead to feelings of guilt and shame, thereby confirming the idea that a tight lid should be kept on one's feelings.

CAT can help carers connect safely with feelings that may otherwise be disavowed, especially those for which they might feel guilty or ashamed, for example, disgust or resentment. Carers need to have experiences of nourishing relational roles, in which they also feel cared for and validated, whether in therapy or from places like organizations supporting carers or support groups, friends and other family members. Through this, they may begin to internalize a different way of noticing their feelings and responding compassionately.

Marva's story

Marva, a black-British woman in her late sixties from the West Indies came to therapy in the context of caring for her husband, Joseph, a man in his early seventies, also from the West Indies. Joseph had been diagnosed with Lewy Body dementia a few years earlier and he required increasing support, including help with dressing, washing, eating and managing incontinence. Joseph often became distressed and asked Marva to sit with him. He was also verbally aggressive towards Marva at times. There was a formal package of care in place, which involved care workers visiting four times a day. Marva found this restrictive as it required her to be at home to let the carers into the house, which meant that she could not go out and socialize as often as she used to. Joseph said he did not like the paid carers, which left Marva feeling guilty for not doing all of the care herself, so she would often help the paid carers do their job when they visited.

Marva had been feeling down and having difficulty sleeping. She described feeling overwhelmed by having so much to think about, including organizing and attending appointments for Joseph, managing his medication, paying bills and managing finances. Marva had several health problems herself, including high blood pressure, arthritis and sciatica, which caused her a lot of pain. Since becoming a carer for Joseph, Marva had been cancelling her health appointments to attend Joseph's appointments with him, even when their adult children had offered to accompany him. Marva was always 'on the go' and she found it very difficult to stop and rest, despite being in a lot of pain.

Marva and Joseph had two adult children together. Marva said that her marriage to Joseph had not been a happy one; he had been unfaithful to her on several occasions, including fathering a child with another woman. Understandably, this led to feelings of resentment on Marva's part, about caring for Joseph when he became unwell. Despite this, she was determined to continue caring for Joseph, seeing it as her 'wifely and Christian obligation'. Marva had stayed married to Joseph because she felt it was her duty, and they had led largely separate lives until Joseph became unwell.

Marva had been referred for therapy in the context of Joseph's dementia deteriorating and her stress levels rising. Upon review, her upbringing was revealed to have been strict and cold. Her parents had been 'Victorian' in their approach to parenting, and Marva would be physically beaten for perceived transgressions. Marva was one of eight children so her mother was often busy. Marva had learned to be self-sufficient from a young age, coming to the UK with one of her siblings as a teenager and working to send money to her parents back in the West Indies. Marva spent much of her life thinking about others, which was driven by her Christian faith, and her strict upbringing in which working hard, being polite and caring were highly valued. Even before becoming a carer for Joseph, Marva regularly visited her elderly or frail relatives and friends, helped others in need and regularly donated money to local hospitals and hospices. At times, Marva felt resentful and angry and thought that she was 'too good' for others, who didn't help her in the same way she helped them, but Marva found it extremely difficult to ask for help, and she declined others' offers of help when they were made. Marva did not want others to see that she was feeling down as she didn't want to worry them, so others often assumed that Marva was fine.

Marva began to understand how her life experiences and the cultural milieu of her upbringing had affected how she lived her life. Like layers of an onion, the different influences or 'voices' from her early life had affected how Marva spoke to herself and others, and what she came to expect from others. Marva realized that she had internalized a demanding, strict way of speaking to herself from her early parental relationships. This, along with the outer layers of the onion – the sociocultural factors such as Victorian and Christian values – led Marva to strive and push herself to work hard and to help others. In CAT terms, Marva was caught in a striving trap.

While it made Marva feel good to help others, it had the unintended downside that her own needs were often overlooked; even her most basic of physical needs such as rest or attending her medical appointments were neglected. In caring for Joseph to the point of self-neglect, Marva also had little time to do the things she had previously enjoyed, like seeing friends or going to the gym. Missing out on socializing caused Marva's mood to decline and neglecting her regular exercise at the gym led to an increase in her physical pain. Marva had no choice but to be self-sufficient as a child, but while this made sense in the context of her early life and felt safer for Marva, it was no longer helpful in the context of being a carer as it left her feeling overwhelmed and struggling to hold the full burden of the caring role. This negatively impacted Marva's sleep and physical symptoms such as high blood pressure.

Along with having to be self-sufficient from a young age, Marva's experience of having her emotional world overlooked, in a busy/overlooking-to-overlooked reciprocal pattern, had taught her to bury and dismiss her feelings. In CAT terms, Marva internalized the busy/overlooking reciprocal pattern towards herself. This allowed her to feel safe by keeping her feelings to herself, rather than expressing them, only to be met with punishment, criticism or disregard. While this worked well when Marva was young, in the caring situation Marva's feelings of resentment bubbled inside, and would sometimes become too much, leading to Marva exploding in anger towards Joseph. Marva would then feel guilty and ashamed, in a way confirming her sense that she should keep her feelings to herself. This is an example of a dilemma, in CAT terms, between Marva either keeping her feelings bottled up and buried, or them exploding out of control. Marva saw that she needed to find a middle ground between these two extremes. This initially started in therapy, where Marva began voicing some of her feelings. Marva made use of assertiveness techniques to help her begin communicating her feelings to others, so she was eventually able to take this outside of the therapy room to begin sharing her feelings with her children and friends.

Figure 7.3: Marva's map

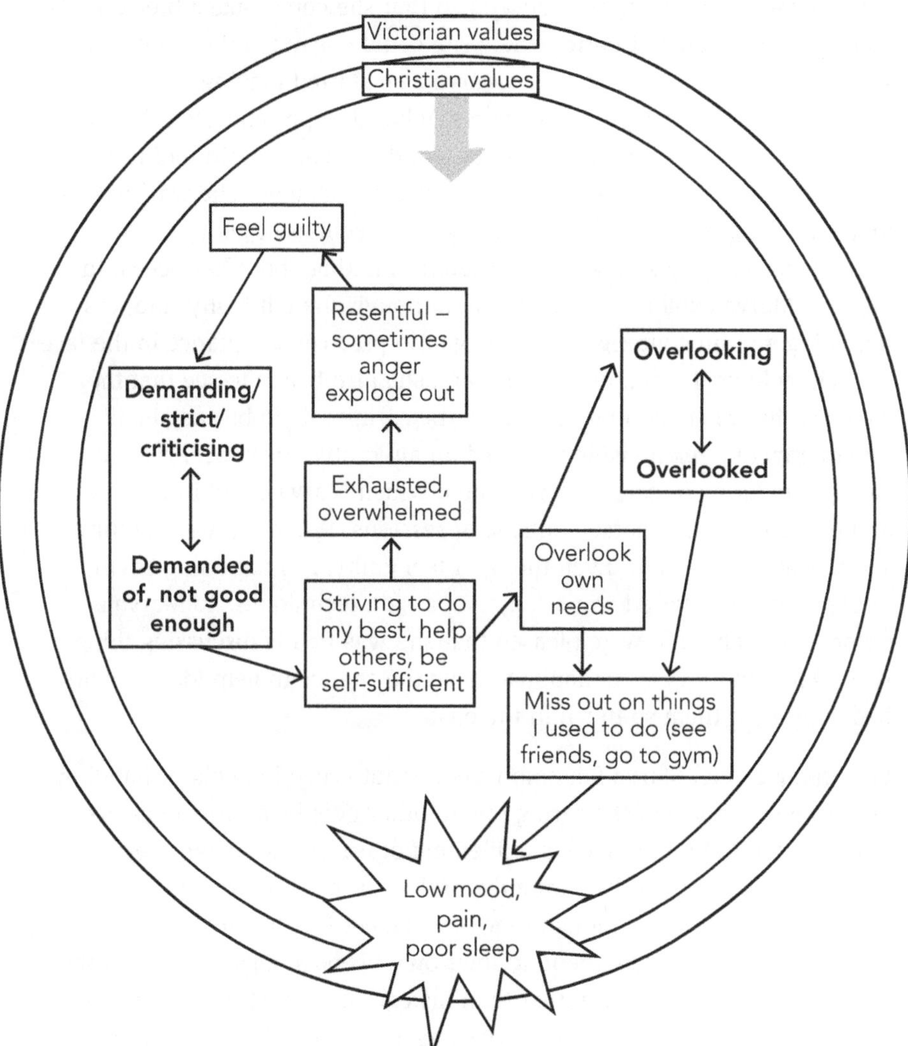

Through understanding the pattern of striving, Marva began to see how she had neglected herself, and the impact that this had on her mood and pain levels. Although difficult, Marva began to make changes to attend more to her own needs, for example leaving the paid carers to do their job without her when they visited, getting a key safe box so that the carers could let themselves in, accepting her children's offers to spend time with Joseph and accompany him to appointments so that she could go to the gym and see her friends. Marva also applied for certain financial benefits that she was eligible for as a carer, which she used to pay a carer to sit with Joseph so that she could take a break or go to the local Carers' Centre, where she could speak to other carers or get free complimentary therapies. Marva also started making changes in her response to Joseph. For example, when Joseph requested things, Marva began to put boundaries in place and sometimes said 'no' to his less reasonable requests. Marva noticed that the changes she was making in acknowledging her own needs brought up feelings of guilt, which was unsurprising as she was so unused to thinking about her needs. In therapy, Marva explored the idea that, although she felt guilty, she was not doing anything wrong and she began to practise acceptance in the face of such feelings. In fact, on the contrary, she also began to see that the changes she was making would allow the caring role to be sustainable. The therapeutic relationship provided an alternative reciprocal role of caring/validating-to-cared for/validated, which Marva could internalize and practise towards herself outside of sessions. When Marva felt guilty, she repeated to herself, 'Even though I feel guilty, I'm not doing anything wrong', and she started using self-compassion techniques. To Marva's surprise, her children were pleased that she was finally discussing things with them, and they were happy to have the chance to help Marva, who had supported them so much in the past.

Like many carers, Marva felt ambivalent about accepting help or handing over some elements of the caring role to other people, even paid carers. Carers often find themselves in a dilemma of feeling as though they *either* have to do all of the caring themselves or have to accept help but feel out of control or as though they have failed. It is helpful to think about how the carer can attend to their own needs alongside those of the person they are caring for, rather than instead of, so that the caring role can be sustainable. As a carer, Marva was also able to learn to accept care and love from her children, as she gradually opened up to them. Marva's experience of caring for someone with whom there is a complex relationship in which there are mixed or contradictory feelings is common. The change of role from partner to carer (or child to carer, or sibling to carer etc.) tends to bring to the fore any difficult patterns or roles that were already there. Often people come to therapy thinking the 'problem' is that their loved one has dementia, when in fact the dementia is just the catalyst that has caused years of complex relational dynamics to manifest or rendered the carer's previous coping strategies unhelpful.

Cultures of care

While some people receive care from relatives at home, others have visits from paid carers, some move to residential care, and others might have a mixture of both care at home and care at a Day Centre, or temporary stays in respite facilities. A large proportion of care home residents in the UK have dementia or memory problems. The move itself to residential care can be extremely disempowering for the person. This can be a particular struggle for people who have previously strived to be self-sufficient and in control, for people with traumatic histories, and for people with experiences of institutional prejudice or abuse. Wherever someone is being cared for, and whomever by, they should receive care that is person-centred, considering their history and identity. Like the 'layers of the onion' that we referred to earlier when thinking about the wider sociocultural context of Marva's life, the wider cultures around care and caring can also be considered. Ideally, personal histories gathered on residents entering residential facilities would encompass an assessment for trauma exposure. This is not generally the case, and nonpharmacological interventions may take a back seat to the convenience and simplicity of relying on behaviour-modifying medications.

Even professionals who are aware of the prevalence and symptomatology of PTSD may not appreciate its potential impact. Given that dementia is a memory disorder that gradually erases one's memories and capacity for self-reflection, some may assume that memories of trauma will also fade and lose their power to upset. The opposite may be true. Traumatic memories can be full of vivid multi-sensory detail but are often fragmented as well; a combination that may be especially frightening for those whose capacity for rational reflection and self-awareness has been compromised by dementia. Recent neuroscience has found that PTSD changes one's brain and nervous system, placing the body and all its senses on constant high alert for perceived threats. This can create intense, instantaneous, fight-flight-freeze responses to stimuli associated with the trauma. These 'triggers' are largely unconscious, and the brain responds to them as though the original traumatic event is taking place in the present, not as something connected with the past. A person who was assaulted years before, for example, may respond to a wrist being taken gently by a nursing assistant as though an assault is occurring in the present and have no awareness that the nervous system is being activated by the original trauma. Such intense reactions can be difficult for trauma survivors under the best of circumstances. When the challenges of cognitive and social impairment are added, it warrants reflection as to the ways dementia might make such experiences even more frightening.

Kitwood (1997) identified a malignant social psychology in which the personhood of people with dementia is undermined in society, particularly in care settings. Kitwood highlighted how things like infantilizing, outpacing, labelling and disempowering people with dementia can undermine their well-being and thwart the provision of person-centred care. Often these things are not done intentionally; they are a symptom of a society that is ageist, in which older people, especially people with dementia, are not seen or are subject to ageist stereotypes. They are also symptomatic of systems in which paid carers are under-trained, under-supported, underpaid and under-staffed; this is at least the case in the UK where we work. Much like the idea of offering care that is trauma-informed, Kitwood emphasized how these malignant cultures can be alleviated when carers embody the spirit of collaboration, validation, negotiation, facilitation, pacing and recognition of a person's identity and values. In CAT terms, this could be thought of as embodying reciprocal roles such as 'validating to validated' or 'negotiating and facilitating to seen and supported'.

Just as the well-being of relatives who are caring for loved ones is a significant factor in the well-being of the person with dementia, the well-being of paid staff is also important. Staff risk burnout, vicarious traumatization, physical and emotional abuse, racism, feelings of helplessness or hopelessness and compassion fatigue. As therapists working in dementia care, we offer support to staff in residential homes using CAT to help contain and offer a helpful framework for making sense of the relational patterns that are being played out. CAT can be used in consultation with staff to help make sense of complex presentations, especially where emotional state shifts occur, which may be confusing and challenging for staff, resulting in splitting and demoralization. Behavioural difficulties are often solely attributed to the client but can be understood as a systemic phenomenon, whereby wider systemic and organizational issues can contribute to the perpetuation of disability and distress. The feelings and emotional reactions generated by the system e.g. staff in a nursing home or community mental health team and carers, can be used to make sense of how individuals are involved in perpetuating unhelpful dynamics and then come up with more helpful alternatives to reduce the level of distress and damage caused by destructive behaviour. CAT can help to make sense of staff, client and system dynamics resulting in the containment of powerful feelings and enabling staff to respond therapeutically and empathically rather than simply reacting to such clients (Ryle & Kerr, 2020). Mapping together can be containing and educative for staff and permits ownership of negative emotions and responses e.g. anger, which may not feel permissible professionally, by locating these in a non-judgemental system of causality.

Summary

CAT is well placed to work therapeutically with older people and their carers by offering a sensitive and versatile relational framework within which to explore psychosocial and intersectional influences, including the legacy of developmental trauma. CAT can take the long view across the lifespan and from generation to generation to explore longstanding relational patterns of carers, both intergenerationally and in self-to-self roles, which influence how the caring role is managed, and where changes for the better can be made for both the person caring and the person being cared for. Adjusting to the changes that come with taking on a caring role or needing to accept care from others, from a previous level of independence, can trigger painful feelings, including those with their legacy in past experiences. CAT offers a sensitive way to make sense of these feelings, within the context of one's life and offers alternatives for living as you care and are cared for.

Chapter 8: Approaching the end – loss, mortality, and new beginnings in later life

Kitty Clark-McGhee and Emma Forde

> *'Since when,' he asked,*
> *'Are the first line and last line of any poem*
> *Where the poem begins and ends?'*
>
> – Seamus Heaney

Introduction: 'Endings' in older age

We are not the first, nor will we be the last, to begin a conversation about 'endings' with the adage that there are only two certainties in life: the certainty of death and the certainty that we will encounter change in our lives. Likewise, it is a well-established truth within therapeutic settings that, in life, we seek to avoid the pain and fear associated with these two certainties, and yet, as we move towards older age, the likelihood and frequency we will encounter the death of a loved one increases; as another adage goes, 'you know you're getting old when you go to more funerals than you do weddings'. In life, we seek out change, often in response to hardships or dissatisfactions, either through adjustments within ourselves or through changes to our environments and relationships with others. But what happens when change is an ending that happens to us? When it has not been invited into our lives nor is it something we can hope to prevent? And what happens when we find ourselves facing that oft-mentioned existential crisis of later life, where we grapple with lost hopes and related feelings of anger, regret, remorse and sadness at what was not possible?

In this chapter, we will be exploring 'endings' in multiple senses of the word, and how you can navigate the challenge of endings in a healthy and healing way. We are putting to one side 'small' endings: the end of a therapy session, a goodbye after a difficult interaction, the denouement of an argument, though these are of course meaningful, and you may find that your reflections lead you to see patterns which parallel the relational tone of larger, more categorical endings and losses. Here, we invite you to explore experiences of death, dying and mourning, as well as more abstract endings that you may find yourself negotiating as an elder; the ambiguous loss that goes hand in hand with health-related changes, either your own or those of someone you care for; and the existential pain of encountering your mortality, which is a healthy but painful dilemma of old age. Throughout, we offer snippets from Maureen's story, a woman in her seventies who was seen by one of the authors for therapy following diagnosis of a debilitating lung condition; her journey illustrates some of the issues under discussion in this chapter. Alongside this, we provide some exercises which we hope will help you to think about, and reflect on, how these issues come up for you in your life.

1. How our 'beginnings' can help us understand our relationship to 'endings'

In CAT, we recognise the importance of looking to our early experiences to understand how endings are managed in later life. Any ending, be that the end of a relationship, the end of a career, the end of a valued familial role, or the end of youth, can come with an associated sense of loss, which can be a source of angst for us all. However, the quality and tone of this angst are quite unique to each of us, shaped by a layering up of our personalities, experiences, and circumstances. As therapists, we first look to early life/childhood as a roadmap for making sense of what a person is finding hard to bear and why. It is no different for understanding how a person relates to the endings they encounter in life, and what, of the resulting feelings, they find most challenging or anxiety-provoking. For example, when we meet a client, we listen out for examples of how childhood experiences of both emotional and physical pain were responded to by caregivers; was there: appropriate care and concern? Fretting? Angry-anxiousness? Frustration? Exasperation? Lesson-learning/telling off? And how were we, often implicitly, encouraged to respond to our pain through what was modelled to us and from the messages we internalised? Were we taught to suffer in silence? Self-criticise? Distract ourselves? Lash out at those around us? Retreat from others to a place of isolation? What early reciprocal roles about distress and suffering were established through these early experiences of relating to distress, and how has that shaped the person's perception of their ability to cope with and manage pain and suffering?

As has been elaborated elsewhere in this book, when these dynamics are a consistent feature of the landscape of our childhood, we not only learn and get familiar with the child-derived role, but we also internalise the parental role about ourselves and others. This is relevant here because early reciprocal roles can get 'activated' when we are navigating an ending of any kind. The changes involved can bring us into contact with core pain that we have learned to guard against through defensive procedures which act to keep us safe from unmanageable feelings and unmet needs. This means that, in response to our struggles in the face of an ending, we might notice ourselves enacting these life-limiting but familiar responses (fretting, frustration, exasperation, angry-anxiousness, distracting, telling off) towards ourselves, since this is our learned response to distress. The corollary is that we are prevented from extending ourselves the care and compassion that, as humans, we need if we are to bear the understandable emotional pain that is the normal human response to an ending, and to find a way to incorporate it into our understanding of ourselves.

Maureen's story

Maureen was referred to the older adult's psychology service during an episode of severe depression. Maureen talked about feelings of fatigue, overwhelm and a sense of being trapped by a chronic lung condition, which affected her mobility and severely restricted her previously independent lifestyle. We talked about Maureen's beginnings to help understand her present; Maureen's father was often absent due to long working hours. Her mother suffered with severe depression for most of Maureen's childhood and Maureen described feeling anxious and as though she were a disappointment to her. Maureen's father died in her teenage years and she understood this loss as being the catalyst for her escape from a family home which she experienced as restrictive; at the age of 17, she left home to work in administration, eventually leading to a busy and glamourous life involving travel abroad and a vibrant, if impersonal, social life. We saw how Maureen's early experiences had left her feeling uncertain about whether others would be responsive to her needs, and a painful impression that those who might offer care will ultimately leave her, alongside a coping idea that when they do leave, she could keep herself safe from painful feelings through self-reliance and running away. Maureen's map began like this:

Figure 8.1: Maureen's map

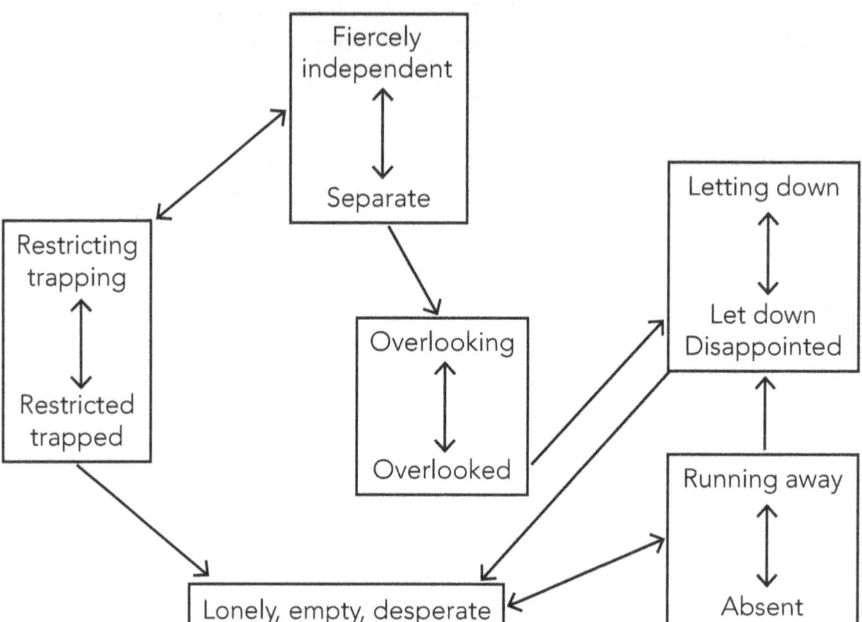

Exercise

Take some time in a quiet place to reflect on the following:

- How do you explain death to yourself?
- Which ideas about death are you most comfortable with?
- What do you believe happens when and after people die?
- Where do your ideas come from?
- How was 'doing grieving' modelled to you growing up?
- As a child, what were the dominant social messages around you about death, dying and mourning?
- What are your first thoughts about how this has shaped the ways you relate to endings and loss?

2. Let's talk about death (and why that feels so hard)

Received wisdom is that death, 'the final taboo', remains a uniquely avoided topic across cultures and that humankind arrives at conversations about death with marked reluctance (Gire, 2014). Fascinatingly, recent research even points to a neurological defense mechanism that hard-wires us to interpret information about our mortality as unreliable or unrelated to ourselves (Sample, 2019). In recognising how harmful this avoidance can be to us both societally and as individuals, strides have been made to redress this; perhaps most notably is the international 'Death Café' movement, a social franchise aiming to increase awareness of death, which started in Hackney, East London, and can now be found in eighty-five countries around the world . Such spaces seek to normalise talking about death processes and their emotional, social and psychological effects. What remains relatively unexplored in published literature, though, is the unique intersection experienced by older adults who face experiences of death, dying and mourning at an increased frequency, alongside an increased sense of closeness to one's mortality, against an ageist social backdrop which at best undermines, and at worst pathologises, processes of grieving. To borrow from grief psychotherapist Julia Samuel, aging has a bad reputation; other life phases are conceptualised as 'development' or progress, whereas the act or process of aging is associated with the image of the slippery slope to death (Samual, 2018). As we age, it becomes harder to avoid awareness of the fragile nature of our lives and our surrounding world. Understandable human anxiety in response to this can be frightening and overwhelming and can lead us to 'block out' or go numb to try to protect ourselves, with the effect that the presence of difficult feelings is denied.

In our work, what we see is just how much people want to talk about death and grief, and that by inviting 'death talk' a person is somehow 'given permission' to talk about their experiences of grief and, often, how this connects with their own life and mortality. By starting to notice and name societal assumptions and their relational consequences, we can begin to undermine the unhelpful dynamics which get in the way of processing loss and its accompanying feelings and prevent us from getting comfortable with the idea of our death, and therefore less fearful of aging/old age.

When someone dies, those around the grieving person can experience feelings of powerlessness, and a related striving procedure to attempt perfect care and rescuing from the terrible circumstances. Those around a person who is grieving may find themselves sharing feelings of helplessness and a sense of overwhelm when it is inevitably not possible to rescue the person from these terrible circumstances. If a person cuts themselves off from their emotions for fear of being overwhelmed by them, others around that person will take that cue and attempt to avoid 'triggering' sadness in the other person. This can lead to a feeling as though both parties (the grieving person and the other/s) are 'treading on eggshells', with the other perceiving that the grieving person might explode/implode/crumble if they are reminded of the loss, and the grieving person feeling as though they are the source of the other person's intense discomfort. 'Avoidance' is a common response to this relational experience; not wanting to talk about it because it feels uncomfortable, so we and others avoid talking about it. In old age, this can be doubled down upon via increased risks of loneliness and isolation, and by generational values such as the 'stiff upper lip', meaning that elders are more likely to be going through grieving processes alone.

Exercise

We find it hard to hold our mortality in mind in the abstract. Take a moment to imagine that you have been told by a medical professional that you are dying. Reflect on the following questions, taking time to notice and pinpoint any discomfort that you experience as you explore this imaginary scenario.

First, imagine the moment that you are told you are dying. Reflect on the following questions:

- How do you feel?
- What do you want to do?
- What is important to you?
- What are you most afraid of?
- What are your wishes in relation to your funeral?
- Who in your life knows this?

Next, imagine the moment of your death. Reflect on the following questions:

- What happens to your body as you die?
- What happens to your mind, or consciousness?
- How are your beliefs and stories about death present in this moment?

Lastly, imagine your funeral. Reflect on the following questions:

- How does it look?
- Are you being buried, cremated or something else?
- Who is there and what are they feeling?
- How are you feeling as you are imagining this loss of self? Sad? Angry? Lonely? Scared?

3. How we negotiate grief, bereavement and mourning in older age

Later life can be a time when a person encounters multiple bereavements. There is an idea that because someone is old, they should expect and therefore 'just get on with' the multiple losses that become more likely as we age. Common expressions like 'they had a good innings' and 'they died a ripe old age' might feel trivialising, or even critical, of a grieving person's emotional pain – moreover, we frequently hear these expressions used about people who died in their seventies; this is striking when we acknowledge that life expectancy in Europe is at least eighty-one, not to mention the advanced older ages of others in the Blue Zones. These expressions are perhaps located in ageist assumptions about worth and youth. These expressions and what they reveal about societal attitudes towards old age contribute to a message that, because death is an expected part of older age, grief should not be complex, complicated or protracted. They aim to offer comfort, and their familiarity to us echoes established 'truths' about death in old age. They also serve to help us avoid complicated, uncomfortable feelings in the face of another person's distress, by giving us something socially acceptable to say. Of course, these sorts of expressions have an important place when encountering another's grief, indeed, sometimes convention is what we have to rely on, such as when we do not know a person so well, when we are carrying our own grief or when the encounter is a very brief one. But, as we are hopefully drawing out, there are also unintended consequences in which an environment is established which lays the ground for feelings of embarrassment, guilt, weakness or shame for struggling with a 'straightforward' death, or else anger or a sense of aloneness/loneliness at how the experience is being minimised by others.

If a person continues to experience intense grief for a length of time beyond that which is 'normal' (six months for adolescents, one year for adults) their experience can be conceptualised as a form of adjustment disorder, despite a troublingly thin evidence base for the diagnosis (Cacciatorie & Frances, 2022). Prevailing models of 'the grief process' are in the mix here. Most well-known is the five stages of grief, attributed to Kubler-Ross, though there are a range of stage-based models with anywhere from three to 12 distinct stages. Crucially, Kubler-Ross's original model, intended as a theory of the experience of dying, has been widely misapplied (Stroebe *et al*, 2017). There is no empirical proof that stage-based models offer a useful, generalisable representation of grief experiences, and they can serve to promote the idea that, if a person cannot recover from and accept the death of a loved one, then they are not successfully adjusting to the reality and are therefore unwell, or mentally ill. We would argue, based on our work with all kinds of people in grief, that a grieving person might eventually find themselves in a place where they can *live with* the pain, and that arriving there is not necessarily a permanent destination nor a journey that takes place over a prescriptive period, despite what prevailing stage-based models, diagnostic manuals and popular beliefs suggest.

The presence of generational ideas about managing and coping with grief and bereavement with a 'stiff upper lip' also need to be considered, along with the related idea that if we or another person is not quietly managing their loss, then they are not coping well enough. This generational message of how to mourn is poorly aligned with therapeutic ideas that adaptive mourning involves 'acknowledging loss and internalising what was lost' (Kerr & Ryle, 2006). Many of us, particularly those of us who were raised according to these sorts of ideas, may not have learned how to mourn in a self-compassionate way. Moreover, for those of us who have a strong inner critic, self-criticism towards one's grief reactions can surface, viewing pain as an intrusion or an irritant that must be eliminated, and keeping us stuck in the tyranny of 'shoulds'. In this way a 'dismissing to dismissed' reciprocal role gets enacted, where we double down on our emotional pain with critical thoughts while at the same time attempting to push away distress so that it is not felt. This means that our distress can bubble up in unexpected, overwhelming ways and reinforce the sense that it is intrusive and unacceptable. These sorts of procedures inhibit our ability to tune into and make sense of our distress, and how it feels in our bodies, and to offer and accept comfort and kindness from ourselves and others in our grief.

Maureen's story (Part 2)

Maureen talked about feeling ashamed and frightened by the new requirement to depend on others, an experience coloured by past hurt of being let down by others throughout her life. We saw how, in the past, her main way of coping with this was to run from difficult situations, people and places, at times even relocating herself, which reinforced a restricting dilemma that she is safe only when not reliant on others. This was quite literally no longer possible, and an alternative 'running from' had begun to emerge in the form of drinking alcohol after abstaining for many years.

We identified a trap, whereby Maureen had learned from a young age to keep her needs and her feelings hidden; an understandable survival strategy in response to the sad reality that those responsible for her needs as a child were unreliable or absent. From this way of relating with others and the world, Maureen had learnt to become intensely self-reliant and to fear needing others, entering into exciting new romantic relationships and friendships, relocating herself, and using her busy job as distraction and distancing from painful feelings. We saw how this helped Maureen to feel safe in her younger years, but contributed to greater loneliness and isolation in the later stages of her life, especially in the face of changes to her physical health. These aspects were added to our map:

Figure 8.2: Maureen's map (Version 2)

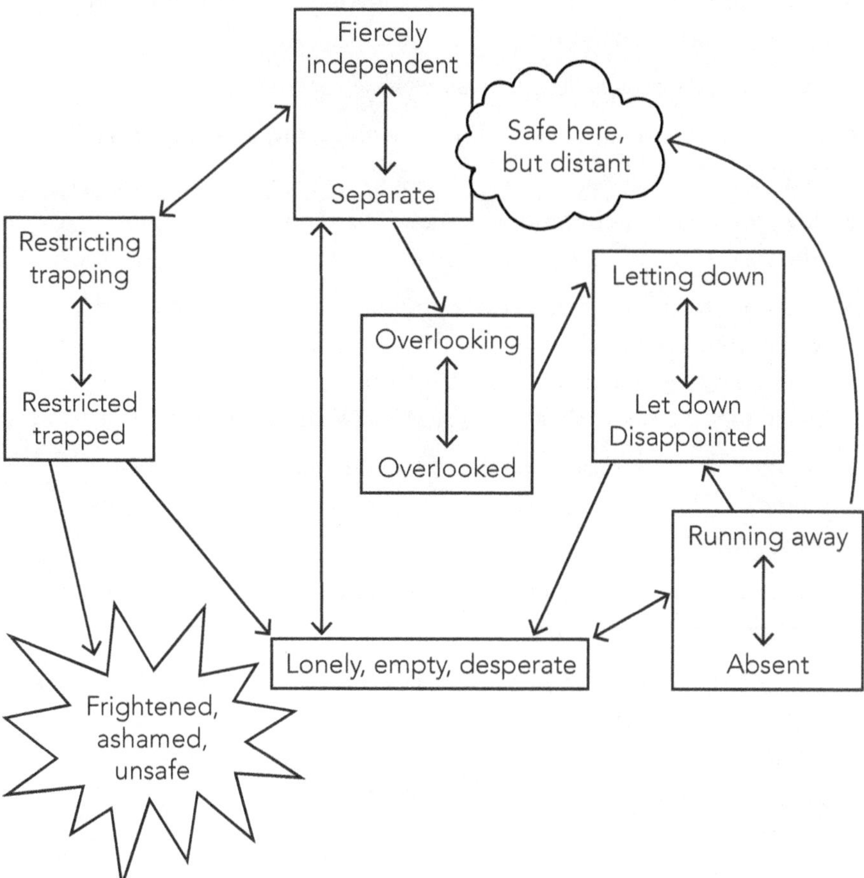

Exercise: Writing a grief story

Storytelling is at the core of the human experience. We make sense of our lives through a narrating process, both internally, within ourselves, and out loud with others in our lives. Opportunities to construct and narrate our evolving grief stories are a core part of recognising all the emotions that we are feeling about our losses.

Start by taking out some paper and a pen, and keep them close by. Now, sit in a place where you feel safe and comfortable. Once you are feeling relaxed, and your mind relatively still, try to connect with the memory of a loved one who has died.

When you feel ready, begin to narrate your story. Alternatively, you might like to experiment with 'mapping' your story with pen and paper; take a look at chapter 3 for some guidance on this. The following questions should also help to guide you:

- What was happening in your life in the moments before you learned of your loved one's death?
- If your loved one was ill, what was this like for you?
- If your loved one died suddenly or unexpectedly, what was this like for you?
- How did the nature of their death, and the time leading up to it, affect you?
- Describe the moment that you learned your loved one had died: where were you? What were you doing at that moment? What were you told by the person who shared the news with you? How did you feel in that moment? What did you think? What did you do?
- How did your loved one's death affect you in the weeks following their death? Were there tasks or responsibilities that required your attention?
- Have you experienced different or new feelings since the time of their death?
- How have you continued to be impacted by their death in the weeks, months, or years since they died?
- When do memories of your loved one come up? How do these memories affect you when they surface?

4. What longstanding procedures might be activated when we encounter loss?

Often, because of an environment of hostility towards talking about grief and death, bereavements that were experienced as children or as younger-age adults remain unprocessed, and we can find the difficult feelings related to these losses coming up in unexpected ways throughout our lives, often about other endings: threats to the ending of a relationship, times of transition which also hold loss (e.g. retirement, becoming a grandparent, becoming a carer or being 'cared for'). As humans, we will always find ways to cope with difficult feelings and, when expressing the sadness of grief is 'off limits' to us, we will, understandably, seek out other ways to cope with the pain, for example:

- Cutting off from one's feelings by keeping too busy to think or feel.
- Relying on alcohol, substances or other numbing practices to blot out pain.
- Either attempting to avoid the pain of loss by entering into intense relationships, or attempting to avoid the pain of loss by avoiding closeness and connection with others.

As a consequence of these problematic procedures, our pain in the face of a loss remains unprocessed and 'live'. Even more so, as an elder, these limited but understandable attempts to keep difficult feelings at bay become harder to sustain – increased isolation, reduced mobility, changes to our physical health, and more frequent encounters with the death of others are all more likely as we move into old age. This makes it even more likely that we will come up against the unresolved pain of past losses, with fewer options available to us for avoidance, distraction and cutting off.

Those of us who repeatedly experienced separation from caregivers when young may have learned to 'detach' ourselves from others and to become more self-reliant so as not to have to depend on unreliable others. The consequences of this can be that feelings of loss (stemming from separation from a caregiver) are repressed or cut off, rather than experienced and resolved. In this way, childhood experiences of unresolved loss become our blueprints for future losses.

For many, what we call an 'anxious-avoidant trap' gets acted out, in which we over-focus on, or worry about, *how* we are grieving (whether it is normal, whether we are depressed or whether there is something 'wrong' with us), and this inhibits us from actually getting to do grieving itself. It may be that this is borne of an environment that pathologises both aging and bereavement and represents the internalisation of a societal-level avoidance of emotional pain, with the consequence that the grieving person is less able to 'get to' feeling sad, bereft, broken-hearted about the absence of the person who died. Interestingly, this trap appears to be a thoroughly modern phenomenon and one that we see less in religious and faith-based communities, possibly because acts of ritual and ceremony serve to take the 'how' out of the grieving person's hands.

Maureen's story (Part 3)

Drawing from Potter's ideas on writing to a part of the self (Potter, 2020), Maureen was invited to write a short letter to the 'fiercely independent' part on our map:

> *Dear fiercely independent me,*
>
> *You helped me to escape at the tender age of seventeen. I travelled the world and had hi-jinx all over the place because of your get-up-and-go. People liked to be around me, I was fun and hard-working, but you also give me a way out - I can pack my bags and off I trot when I need to. I suppose it is 'fierce' because I needed it to be - when people let you down, you can keep on and look after yourself. Now I feel all mixed up because I have lost this part of me - I am not sure who I am if I can't be independent and look after myself. What do I do now that I'm trapped at home with this horrible illness?*

This short exercise brought to the surface greater ambivalence towards 'fierce independence' than Maureen had previously been in touch with. It enabled her to take a tentative step towards the feelings of loss and grief that she had been experiencing in relation to the changes in her elder years. With time we named a place on the map which she called 'a bit of caring / a little bit cared for', which manifested in her tolerating help from physiotherapy and occupational health staff to increase her physical comfort, as well as keeping in better touch with one of her oldest friends, her brothers and her niece and nephew. We added this exit to the map:

Figure 8.3: Maureen's map (Version 3)

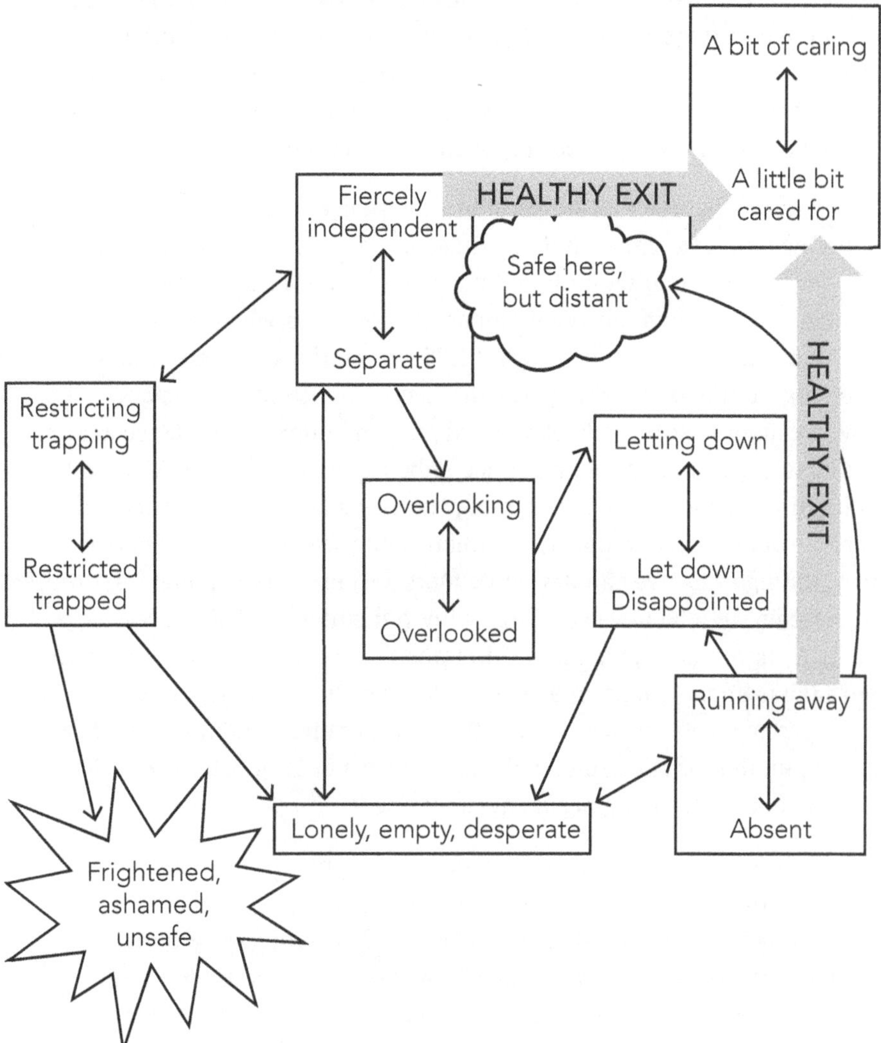

5. Negotiating endings: how we can re-story aging, loss and change in the context of later life

As others in this book have described, we can use CAT ideas to make sense of the unique challenges and transitions that we each encounter in later life and what they mean to us as individuals. Crucially, these ways of making sense invite possibilities of change for the better which, in the face of problematic social and cultural expectations of aging, can be powerful acts of rebellious hoping. All too often, our dominant procedures relating to old age are grounded in feelings of hopelessness and despair, and an idea of being undeserving ('it's too late to change', 'if only I'd done something years ago', 'others need this more than me'). To some extent, this prejudice transcends global geography and culture, since urbanisation, industrialisation and, later, post-industrial society are global phenomena which have served to shape old age as a societal burden. That there are many benefits of an aging society seems beyond our collective ZPD.

We all know that the fullness of human existence includes pain and suffering, and yet, since we find pain so abhorrent, we seek to eliminate it by avoiding it, cutting it off and pushing it away. This is a natural human instinct, driven by evolutionary responses to what we perceive as threatening, harmful or dangerous. However, the snag here is that avoiding/cutting off/pushing away are temporary solutions to pain, which cannot ever be truly eliminated from the human experience and which, sooner or later, will resurface to be experienced again. More to the point, this instinctive survival strategy keeps us from learning that we are capable of attending to our pain without futile attempts to eliminate it and that, through this, we can develop a more sustainable relational response to our pain, in which we can 'bear with' our suffering. The process of adjustment to major life, and death, transitions is not a swift one, despite our understandable human ache for it to be so; it is almost always the case, perhaps with dementia and other degenerative conditions as a key exception, that physical/literal change happens at far greater speed than the emotional reckoning occurring alongside it.

As we have talked about, a common experience among grieving people is a sense of embarrassment or shame in feeling the way they do; this speaks to a pervasive social culture which positions sadness, especially grief, as embarrassing or even shameful and sends a message to those who are grieving that they should stay silent in their grief. An important antidote to this unhealthy (repressive) societal-level relational response, and something that repeatedly comes up as a feature of people's grief process, is the importance of finding a connection with others who are experiencing grief. We have heard this described by clients as though they have become members of a 'secret club' where they can talk openly about having lost someone. This brings with it a sense of relief, alongside an impression that this kind of talk is not permissible in everyday interactions. For elders, this can present a unique challenge though; it may be harder to access these kinds of networks if you are also grappling with reduced mobility or physical freedom as you age, and the effects of COVID may have exacerbated this too.

Beyond this, throughout life, we face many endings, and to survive these we will draw on the procedures that we have developed and honed since our earliest years. As has been illustrated elsewhere in this book, as an elder though, the nuts and bolts of these relied-upon procedures become harder to maintain, owing to physical, cognitive or social changes that are a part of the landscape of older age. This means that you might find yourself facing an ending without your usual coping strategies; whether these ways of coping might be categorised as 'functional' or 'dysfunctional', they have enabled you to survive up until this point, and to no longer be able to draw upon these to reliable effect can be experienced as overwhelming and frightening. Part of the challenge here is learning to distinguish between feelings relating to an ending and, therefore, a possible new beginning, and feelings relating to the end, in other words, to your mortality and inevitable death. These different sets of emotional responses are related but separate and can get tangled up in each other, particularly in older age, when we tend to experience more deaths of loved ones and more changes in our physical selves. This can make the lifetime's habit of avoiding thinking about our death untenable and, understandably, can also leave us feeling deeply overwhelmed and stuck, unable to see a way forward in the face of change.

This final mapping exercise builds on the concept of mindful self-compassion, introduced in Chapter 2. It will encourage you to acknowledge and explore with self-compassion the range of emotions that you feel about loss and endings. You can use this exercise in different ways: either to explore your emotions about a specific bereavement or loss or, to explore your emotions about your mortality and death. In this exercise, we particularly invite you to experiment with mapping your self-to-self emotional experience and the dialogue between your feelings; Chapter 3 offers a rich guide if you feel unsure about mapping.

Exercise: Mapping the emotional landscape of endings

Start by taking out some paper and a pen and keeping it close by. Sit in a place where you feel safe and comfortable. Once you are feeling relaxed, and your mind relatively still, take a moment to identify whether you will use this exercise to explore your emotions about a specific bereavement or loss, or your own mortality and death.

Imagine that each of your emotions is like a 'lily pad' (a discrete state of being). On your paper, write down each of the emotions that you are aware you are feeling when you are thinking about this ending. →

Some emotions may come easily (sadness, longing, tiredness, helplessness), while others may feel more fleeting, uncomfortable or unwanted (guilt, anger, hatred, relief). Remind yourself that there are no wrong feelings here, only noticing and naming what is there. Each of these lily pads represents different relational parts of yourself and each part has different hopes and needs.

Once you have your 'lily pads' on your page, take each one in turn, and reflect on the following:

- What thoughts does this part of you have about this ending?
- How does this part of you feel about this ending?
- Where can you most connect with this part in your body? Where can you most strongly locate it?
- What is this part of you hoping for? What does it want? What does it need?

Next, draw out one final lily pad and write something like 'wise, loving compassion' inside it. This part of you has unconditional positive regard and warmth for the full range of your emotions. It cares for you deeply and holds your best interests uppermost. Imagine that this part is listening to each of the other parts of you, represented by the lily pads. Reflect on the following:

- What does the wise compassionate part want to say to each of the other parts?
- What does it see that each of the other parts needs? (to hear, to feel, to do)?

Maureen's story (Part 4)

While Maureen was in therapy, at about session eighteen of twenty-four, she learned that her lung condition was a terminal one and that she would require palliative care in the foreseeable future. Maureen expressed deep pain and anger at the illness taking control of her life, alongside intense regret at the loss of her hoped-for future. Together in therapy we noticed a mutual pull akin to the 'running away' part on the map, in the face of the finality of the ending ahead of us, which felt, at times, as though it was 'too big' for us to negotiate without becoming overwhelmed and then trapped. We saw that this avoidance was rooted in a fear that talking about (negotiating) Maureen's mortality would give rise to an unmanageable grief. Relatedly, our remaining sessions were grounded in an intention of staying with the layers of grief in Maureen's present experience, as much as we could, and to offer an ending to the therapy that was more connected to, less retreating from, feelings. Maureen received palliative care and died at home, as was her wish. Until her death, she remained in close contact with loved ones.

Summary

In this chapter, we have explored endings, in multiple senses of the word – from experiences of death and mourning to the presence of loss and change in older age, to increased awareness of one's mortality. Endings are central within therapeutic understandings of CAT since their legacy informs so much of how we learn to cope with loss throughout life, for better or worse. We hope that the exercises in this chapter have helped you to begin to reflect on some of the dilemmas that can arise about endings and to offer new insights and ideas for how to manage the inevitable challenge of endings in healthy and healing ways in later life.

Afterword

Later life brings many opportunities for emotional growth and developmental strengths, including increased acceptance and focus on life in the here and now. Aging, as with other life stages, has its strengths and challenges, with ongoing scope for learning and change. We set out to offer ideas to support self-reflection and develop relational awareness within the context of aging, drawing on the different voices and experiences of the authors in the book, along with research. Whether you are in your later years yourself or supporting someone in theirs, we hope that these different perspectives have offered new understandings and show that it is possible to change long-held and unhelpful patterns, thereby improving emotional well-being in later life. If we open ourselves to developing our inner resources for managing difficult experiences, living well is possible, right to the end of our lives.

These ideas and strategies will take practice, so whenever you falter, remind yourself why you are doing this. If you are supporting someone else to make changes, hold onto hope when theirs may falter. Change takes time, not least when it comes to deeply held lifelong relationship patterns. Watch out for unhelpful patterns when challenges arise and please do not give up. These strategies are designed to be flexible, and change is an ongoing process – our stories continue to unfold as each new day brings new challenges and insights for managing these. Remember, please seek professional help if difficulties become unmanageable and beyond what is possible to manage alone or with help from your personal support circles. Celebrate the exceptions and successes. Nurture your skills of acceptance and self-compassion. Being in the moment is precious – make the most of it now. And if you have gone on this journey of self-development alone, please use new relational insights to reach out to others and sustain supportive connections to keep you going.

CAT as a therapeutic model continues to develop, and its essence is an ongoing dialogue of new understandings, insights and research. We close with a reminder of CAT's central theory being the social formation of our minds. It sees each person as coming into being through different relationships and interactions with others, within different social and cultural contexts. In these fractured times, where relationships can feel so polarized, with every person out for themselves and rates of isolation soaring, the model urges us all to remember that we all have a responsibility to ensure everyone, across generations, can flourish. Growth and development are possible and it is never too late to change.

Appendix 1: The Psychotherapy File

This Appendix is to help us to understand ourselves better so we can begin to sort out our difficulties. We all have one life, which is ours to live. What has happened to us in our lives helps to make us the way we are now. What we have been through sets up ways of thinking, feeling and doing which we repeat over and over again as sort of a pattern in our lives.

Sometimes, difficult situations and events in our lives start up patterns of thinking, feeling and behaving, which may help at the time but which later may become hurtful to us. We can therefore get on better with our lives if we can break these patterns and learn to do things differently. This can be hard because we have had the patterns for so long.

- The first step in sorting out your difficulties is to identify the hurtful patterns which you have in your life.
- The second step is to see when they happen in your life now.
- The third step is to work at trying to do things in another way.

In this way, you can begin to have more control or say in your life and more happiness.

Remember:

- The patterns arise because of what has happened to us in our lives.
- They are how we got by in difficult times.
- It is not because we are bad or stupid.
- We don't have to keep doing them if we learn to see what is happening.
- By changing the way we do things, we can learn to control our behaviour.
- When we change, the way other people behave towards us may also change.
- It is possible for things to change.

Keeping a diary of the way you feel and what you do

We can begin to sort out our moods and difficult behaviour by learning to identify when they start and what sets them off. Start keeping a diary, every day, if possible. Think about when an unwanted mood or behaviour happened. Try to write down what you were *feeling* and *thinking* and what was *happening* at the time.

We can talk about this in our time together. You can also talk about it with anyone else you would like to.

Thinking about patterns

This page will help us to work out your patterns. These questions will help us work out traps you can get into which go round and round in a hurtful way. Please mark yes or no.

1. Are you afraid of hurting other peoples' feelings?	yes / no
■ *If yes* – Do you hide your feelings and needs inside when you are with other people?	yes / no
2. Do you get fed up with yourself?	yes / no
■ *If yes* – Do you think you can't do things very well?	yes / no
3. Are you worried that you may not be good enough for other people?	yes / no
■ *If yes* – Do you try to please people who you are with?	yes / no
4. Do you get worried when you go out?	yes / no
■ *If yes* – Does this stop you going out?	yes / no
5. Do you feel worried that you are not very good at being with people?	yes / no
■ If yes – Does this sometimes make it hard for you to be friendly?	yes / no
6. Do you sometimes feel you are no good as a person?	yes / no
■ *If yes* – Do you think that you will not be able to get what you need or want?	yes / no
■ *If yes* – Do you think you can't have what you need or want because if you do …	yes / no
■ … you will be told off?	yes / no
■ … people close to you will go away?	yes / no
■ … people will not like you?	yes / no
■ … it won't last?	yes / no
■ … you think you are weak and so you must not let yourself have what you want?	yes / no

More questions about patterns

Sometimes, the way we have come to see things means that we live as if there is not much choice in what we can do. In this way, we can make things harder than they need to be for ourselves.

If we can work out how this happens in your life, we can try to find other ways of doing things which will give you more choices and give you more say in your life.

Do you have any of these patterns?

I must keep my feelings inside of me. If I do not, other people will not like me.	yes / no
I must keep my feelings inside or I will hurt other people.	yes / no
If I am told I must do something, then I don't want to.	yes / no
If I am told I must not do something, then I want to do it.	yes / no
If I get what I want, I feel as if I have done something wrong.	yes / no
If I don't get what I want, I feel cross and unhappy.	yes / no
I have to keep things very, very neat and tidy.	yes / no
If I don't I am scared there will be a terrible mess.	yes / no
With other people, I feel like either I get very close but feel scared I will be hurt or I keep well away and feel lonely.	yes / no
With other people, I feel like *either* I stick up for myself and nobody likes me *or* I give in and get put on by others and feel cross and hurt.	yes / no
With other people, I feel like *either* I feel very, very safe and very, very happy *or* I am being very, very cross with them and wanting to be in a fight with them.	yes / no
I think I am better than other people or else I feel they are better than me.	yes / no
With other people, either I am very close but feel taken over *or* I stay in charge but feel far away and feel lonely	yes / no
When I'm close to someone, either I have to do what they say or they have to do what I say.	yes / no

More patterns

Sometimes we say 'I want to have a better life or I want to change the way I behave BUT…' Maybe this is because other people in our lives have stopped us from having good things for ourselves. Sometimes it seems that we stop ourselves from having good things.

It is helpful to learn to see how this pattern may be stopping you from getting on with your life, so that you can begin to get a better life and keep it. These questions will help us work it out:

Do you ever feel that you are stopped from doing good things or having good things because you are afraid of what other people might say or do?	yes / no
Do you ever feel that you are stopped from doing good things or having good things by something inside yourself telling you that you are not good enough to have them?	yes / no

Remember:

All these patterns arise because of what has happened to us in our lives. They are how we got by in difficult times. It is not because we are bad or stupid. We don't have to keep doing them now that we are learning to see what is happening.

By changing the way we do things, we can learn to control our behaviour. When we change, the way other people behave towards us also changes. It is possible for things to change.

Difficult moods that come in a rush

Some people find it very difficult to keep control over their behaviour because of times when things feel very difficult and different from usual.

Is any of this like you?

How I feel about myself and others can change suddenly, in a rush.	yes / no
Sometimes I get in a mood when I have very, very strong feelings that I can't control.	yes / no
Sometimes I get in a mood when I feel muddled and have no feelings.	yes / no
Sometimes I can be in a mood when I feel very, very cross and angry with myself and want to hurt myself.	yes / no
Sometimes I get in a mood when I feel that others are going to let me down or hurt me.	yes / no
I can get in a mood when I feel very, very angry and hurtful to others.	yes / no
Sometimes the only way I can cope with confusing feelings is to blank them off, rub them out, and feel very far faraway from others.	yes / no

More questions about strong, upsetting moods that may come in a rush

Do you ever feel strongly like this?

Put in more words or cross out if you want to…

No feelings, far away	yes / no
Out of control, very cross, rage	yes / no
Very special, looking down on others	yes / no
Let down by life and other people	yes / no
Playing others up	yes / no
Clinging to others, afraid of being left alone	yes / no
Very busy, can't think or feel	yes / no
Upset, all in a muddle, feeling scared	yes / no
Feeling wonderfully cared for, very happily close to another	yes / no
Not liked, not wanted, left alone	yes / no
Very cross with myself, thinking I'm no good	yes / no
Helpless and needy, waiting for others to make it all right for me	yes / no
Wanting what other people have, wanting to hurt and upset them	yes / no
Looking after myself and others	yes / no
Hurting myself and hurting other people	yes / no
Feeling cross about doing what other people say I must do	yes / no
Hurt and made to feel small by others	yes / no
Safe in myself and able to be close to others	yes / no
Very cross with myself for things I can't do or mistakes I make	yes / no
Very cross with others for things they can't do or mistakes they make	yes / no
Very scared of others	yes / no

→

Do you get any other very strong moods? Please write below	yes / no

1. For more information, see www.unitedforallages.com/
2. There is a theory in psychology of the 'replacement child' – one who is somehow never good enough and the earlier child, who might have been over idealised, is the favoured.
3. This discussion of voices draws heavily on Ryle and Kerr (2020) and Leiman (2002).
4. Writing 'no send letters' can be a helpful therapeutic exercise in which you write a letter to someone you don't feel you can talk directly to – perhaps a family member, someone you've had difficulties with, but also including people who may have since died. The idea is that you write about your feelings openly – so they're 'out there' – which can help to process them rather than them keeping you stuck, without the letter actually been sent.
5. See https://deathcafe.com/

Appendix 2: The Psychosocial Checklist

The social and political circumstances of our lives can have as much if not more influence on how we feel as our own individual histories and experiences. It can sometimes help us make sense of how we feel if we recognise the broader social and cultural context that influences us.

Please tick the boxes that you feel apply to you:

Aspects of myself or my life that I feel unhappy about, disadvantaged by or in which I feel 'different' from other people.

	Applies strongly	Applies	Does not apply	Comments
1. Mental Health Issues				
2. Ethnicity				
3, Class (eg. money I status I job)				
4. Housing problems or homelessness				
5. Education				
6. Religion				
7. Culture				
8. Being female / being male				

→

	Applies strongly	Applies	Does not apply	Comments
9. Sexual orientation				
10. Physical disabilities				
11. Ill Health				
12. Marital / family situation				
13. Age				
14. The law				
15. Nationality / refugee status				
16. Politics				
17. Personal appearance				
Other – please specify				

Appendix 3: Glossary of Key CAT terms

Dilemmas: Patterns where possible actions are polarized – Either-Or, If-Then – with no middle or balanced option.

Goodbye letters: These are typically exchanged at the end of therapy as a means of summing up and evaluating what has been achieved and what remains to be worked on.

Maps: Visual diagrams illustrating the relational patterns and procedures that maintain them, to offer a way to see where alternatives might be possible.

Reciprocal roles (RR): A stable pattern of interaction (combining action, memory, feelings and expectations), which is developed in relationships with caregivers in early life, and which influences current patterns of relating with oneself and others. We often expect what is familiar to us, and seek out what is familiar, even when it might be harmful. It is bringing these into conscious awareness and understanding that offers the possibility of questioning their usefulness in our lives and then do things differently if needed.

Reformulation letter: These are typically exchanged as a verbal summary of the reasons a person has come into therapy, naming the particular relational patterns to be worked on and reflections on how these manifest within the therapy relationship.

Snags: Patterns where legitimate and appropriate goals are abandoned or undone either because of the assumed attitudes of others or because of irrational guilt.

Target problems (TPs): Target problems are developed from presenting complaints and issues. They are agreed as the problems that therapy will address, typically turning these into something doable, manageable and preferably couched in interpersonal language. For example, feeling depressed might be 'I don't know how to express my feelings and get my needs met, yet'.

Target problem procedure (TPPs): A verbal description of the patterns and sequences that form each target problem. By identifying these – in the form of reciprocal roles, traps, snags, and dilemmas – insights can be developed into how problems are maintained and how different reactions, responses and actions may be taken to break or change unhelpful patterns.

Traps: A self-reinforcing pattern of thought and behaviour, for example a negative belief generates a form of action which produces consequences that are seen to confirm the belief.

References

AARP (2016) The longevity economy: How people over 50 are driving economic and so*cial value in the us [online]. Avail*able at: www.aarp.org/content/dam/aarp/home-and-family/personal-technology/2016/09/2016-Longevity-*Economy-AARP.*pdf (accessed March 2024).

ACAT (undated) CAT Evidence Base [online]. Available at: www.engage.acat.org.uk/cat-evidence-base/ (accessed March 2024).

Age *UK (2018) All the Lonely People: Loneliness in l*ater life [online]. Available at: www.ageuk.org.uk/latest-press/articles/2018/october/all-the-lonely-people-*report/ (accessed Ma*rch 2024).

Allers CT, Benjack KJ & Allers NT (1992) Unresolved childhood sexual abuse: Are older adults affected? Journal of Counseling & Develop*ment 71 14-17.*

Amano, T., & Toichi, M. (2014). Effectiveness of the on-the-spot-EMDR method for the treatment of behavioral symptoms in patients with severe dementia. Journal of EMDR Practice and Research, 8(2), 50–65. https://doi.org/10.1891/1933-3196.8.2.50

Baltes MM & Cartensen LL (1996) The Process of Successful Aging. Ageing and Society, i6, 397-422

Baltes PB & Baltes MM (1993) Successful Aging: Perspective*s from the behavioural sciences (V*ol 4). Cambridge University Press.

Baltes PB (1997) On the incomplete architecture of human ontogency: Selection, optimization, and compensation as foundation of d*evelopmental theory. American Psycholo*gist 52 (4) 366–380. doi: 10.1037/003-066X.52.4.366

Baron J, Asch DA, Fagerlin A, et al (2003) Effect of assessment method on the discrepancy between judgments of health disorders people have and do not have: a web study. Med Decis Making 23 *(5) 422–34.*

Beck AT, Rush AJ, Shaw BF & Emery G (1979) Cognitive Therapy of Depression. New York: Guilford Press.

Bell S (2019) Happiness Across the Life Span: Not a Slippery Slope after all [online]. USC Dornsife. Available at: https://dornsife.usc.edu/news/stories/people-get-happier-as-they-age/ (accessed March, 2024).

Blazer *DG & Hyb*els CF (2014) Depression in later life: Epidemiology, assessment, impact, and treatment. In: IH Gotlib & CL Hammen (Eds.) Handbook of Depression (3rd ed., pp*429-447). Guildford Press.*

Bowlby J (1979) The Making and Breaking of Affectional Bonds. Tavistock Publications Ltd: London.

*Braveman P, Eger*ter S & Williams DR (2011) The Social Determinants of Health: Coming of Age. Annual Review of Public Health 32 1 381-398.

Bromberg P (1998) Standing in the Spaces. Brighton: Psychology Press.

Buettner D (2012) The Blue Zones, Sec*ond Edition: 9* lessons for living longer from the people who've lived the longest. National Geographic.

Bunting M (2004) Willing Slaves: How the overwork culture is ruling our lives. Harper Co*llins.*

Butler J & Ciarrochi J (2007) Psychological acceptance and quality of life in the elderly. Qual Life Res 16 607–615.

Cacciatorie J & Frances A (2022) DSM-5-TR turns normal grief into a mental disorder. The Lancet Psychiatry 9 (7).

Calouste Gulbenkian Foundation and the Centre for Aging Better (2019) Navigating Later Life Transitions: an evaluation of emotional and psychological interventions [online]. Available at: https://ageing-better.org.uk/resources/later-life-transitions-evaluation-emotional-psychological-inter*ventions (accessed March 2024).*

Campbell-Sills L, Barlow DH, Brown TA, Hofmann SG (2006) Effects of suppression and acceptance on emotional responses of individuals with anxiety and mood disorders. Behav*iour Research and Therapy 44 1251–*1263.

Cantacuzino M (2022) Forgiveness: An exploration. Simon & Shuster: UK.

Carers UK (2019) State of Caring report. Available at: https://www.carers*uk.org/media/khgk*b3fs/state-of-caring-2019-report.pd*f (accessed Apr 2024).*

*Carers Worldwide Imp*act Report (2020) Impact Report 2020 [online]. Available a*t: https://carersworldwide.org/images/publications/*Carers-Worldwide-Impact-Report-2020.pdf (accessed March 2020).

Carstensen L (2021) Socioemotional selectivity theory: the role of perceived endings in human motivation. Gerontol*ogist 61 (8) 1188–1196.*

Carstensen L (2022) The New Map of Life: A report from the Stanford Center on Longevity [online]. Available at: https://longevity.stanford.edu/the-new-map-of-life-report/ (accessed March 2024).

Carstensen LL & Fredrickson BL (1998) Influence of HIV status and age on cognitive representations of others. Health Psychology 17 (6) 494–503. doi:10.1037//0278-6133.17.6.494.

Carstensen LL (1992) Social and emot*ional patterns in adulthood: Support for socio***em**otional selectivity theory. Psychology and Aging 7 (3) 331–338. doi:10.1037//0882-7974.7.3.331.

Carstensen LL (1993) Motivation for social contact across the life span: A theory of socioemotion*al selectivity. In: JE Jacob (Ed.) Nebraska Sym***po**sium on Motivation: 1992, Developmental perspectives on motivation (Vol. 40, pp. 209–254). University of Nebraska Press.

Carstensen LL (2006) *The influence of a sense of time on human development.* Science 312 (5782) 1913–1915. doi:10.1126/science.1127488.

*Carstensen LL, Turan B, Scheibe S, Ram N, Ersner-Hershfield H, Samanez-Larkin GR, Brooks KP & Nesselro*ade JR (2011) Emotional experience improves with age: Evidence based on over 10 years of experience sampling. Psychology and Aging 26 (1*) 21–33. doi:10.1037/a0021285.*

Centre **fo**r Aging Better (2022) State of Ageing [onlin*e]. Avai*lable at: https://ageing-better.org.uk/state-of-ageing (accessed March 2024).

Cernik L (2022) 'I've always thrown myself into work, now it keeps me alive: the over-65s forced to join the "the great unretirement"'. 14 September. The Guardian.

Charles *ST, Reynolds CA & Gatz M (2001)* Age-related differences and change in posi*tive and negative affect over 23 years. Journal* of Personality and Social Psychology 80 (1) 136–151. https://doi.org/10.1037/0022-3514.80.1.136.

Cheng ST & Yim YK (2008) Age differences in forg*iveness: The role of future time perspective.* Psychology and Aging 23 (3) pp676-680. doi: 10.1037*/0882-7974.23.3.676.*

Chopik WJ, Newton NJ, Ryan Lh, Kashdan TB & Jarden AJ (2019) Gratitude across the life span: Age differences and links to subjec*tive well-being. The Journal of Positive Psychology, 14 (3) 292-302. doi: 101080/1743976.2017.*1414296.

Clare L & Shakespeare P (2004) Negotiating the impact of forgetting: Dimensions of resistance in task-oriented conversations between people with dementia and their partners. Dementi*a 3 (2) 211-232.*

Connors MH, Seeher K, Teixeira-Pinto A, Woodward M, Ames D & Brodaty H (2020) Dementia and caregiver burden: A three-year longitudinal study. International Journal of Geriatric Psychiatry 35 (2) 250-258.

Criado Perez C (2019) Invisible Wome*n: Exposing d*ata bias in a world desig*ned for men. Chatto and Windus: London.*

*Cribb J et al (2023) In*stitute of Fiscal Studies. The gender gap in pensi*on saving [online]. Available at: https://ifs.org.uk/publica*tions/gender-gap-pension-saving (accessed March 2024).

Davison, EH, Pless Kaiser, A., Spiro, A., Moye, J., King, L.A., & K*ing, D.W. (2016). From late-onset stress symptomatology to later-adulthood trauma* reengagement in ageing combat veterans: Taking a broader view. Gereontologist, 56(1): 14-21.

Davison, EH. (2006). Late-life *emergence of early life* trauma. Research on Aging, 28(1): 84-114.

Dening KH, Greenish W, Jones L, Mandal U & *Sampson EL (2012) Barr*iers to providing end-of-life care for people with dement*ia: A whole-system qualitative study. BMJ Supportive and Palliative Care 2 (2) 103–107.*

Dicks H (1967) Marital Tensions: Clinical studies towards a psychological the*ory of interaction. Routledge.*

Dodd C (2018) 'Life keeps evolving: six ways to have a happy retirement'. 6 October. The Guardian.

Em*bracing Carers (2020). The global carer w*ell-being index. Who cares for carers? Perspectives on COVID-19 pressures and lack of support [online]. Available at: https://www.embracingcarers.com/wp-co*ntent/uploads/Global-***Ca**rer-Well-Being-Index-Report_FINAL.*pdf (accessed Apr 2024).*

*English T & Carstensen LL (2014) Selective narrowing of social ne*tworks across adulthood is associated with improved emotional experience in daily life. International Journal of Behavioral Development 38 (2) 195–202. do*i:10.1177/0165025413515404.*

Erikson E (1950) Childhood and So*ciety. Second edition. Norton: New York.*

Erikson EH (1950) Childhood and society. WW Norto*n & Co.*

Erikson EH (1959) The problem of ego identity. Psychological Issues 1 101–164.

Erikson EH (1982) The Life Cycle Comple*ted. A Review. WW Norton & Co.*

Erikson EH (1984) Reflection on the last stage – and the first. Psychoanalytic Study of the Child 39 155–165.

Erikson EH, Eri*kson J & Kivnick H (***198**6) Vital Involvement in *Old Age. Nortoq, New York.*

*Evans E et al (2019) Nav*igating later life transitions: an evaluation of emotional and psychological interventions. Report for Calouste Gulbenkian Foundation, UK branch.

Felitti VJ, Anda RF, Nordenberg D, Williamson DF, Spitz AM, Edwards V, Koss *MP & Marks JS (1998) Rel***ati**onship of childhood abuse and household dysfunction to many of the leading causes of death in adults. The Adverse Childhood Experiences (ACE) Study. Am J Prev Med. 14 (4) 245-58. doi: 10.1016/s0749-3797(98)00017-8. PMID: 9635069.

Fennel (1999) Overcoming Low Self-Esteem, 2nd Edition: A self-help guide using cognitive behavioural techniques. Overcoming Books.

Fulmer T, Paveza G, Vandeweerd C, Guadagno L, Fairchild S, Norman R, Abraham I & Bolton-Blatt M (2005) Neglect assessment in urban emergency de*partments and con*fir**m**ation by an expert clinical team. Journals of Gerontology. Series A, Biological Sciences and Medical Sciences 60 (8) 1002-1006.

Fung HH & Carstensen LL (2004) Motivat*ional changes in response to blocked goals and foresho***rt**ened time: Testing alternatives *to socioemotional selectivity the*ory. Psychology and Aging 19 (1) 68–78. doi:10.1037/0882-7974.19.1.68.

Fung HH, Lai P & Ng R (2001) Age differences in social preferences among Taiwanese and Mainland Chinese: The role of perceived time. Psychology and A**g**ing 16 (2) 351–356. doi:10.1037//0882-7974.16.2.351.

Gay P (1988) Freud: A life for our time. WW Norton & Co: Londo*n.*

George LK, Blazer DF, Winfield-Laird I, Leaf PJ & Fischbach RL (1988) Psychiatric disorders and mental health service use in later life: evidence from the Epidemio*logic Catchment Area Progra*m. In: J Brody and G Maddox (Eds.) Epidemiology and Aging: An international perspect*ive (pp. 189-219). Springer.*

*Germer C (2009) The Mindful P*ath to Self-Compassion: Freeing yourself from destructive thoughts and emotions. Guildford Press.

Gibran K (1923) The Prophet. Alf*red A Knopf.*

*Gibson RC (1995) Promo*ting successful and productive aging in minority populations. In: LA Bond, SJ Cutler *& A Grams (Eds.) Promoting Succ*essful and Productive Aging (pp 279-288). Thousand Oaks, CA: Sage.

Gilbert P (2009) The Compassionate Mind. Little, Brown *Book Group (pp83-84).*

Gilbert P, Braehler C, Cree M, Gale C, Gillespie C et al (2010) Training Our Minds In, with and for Compassion an Introduction to Concepts and Compassion-Focused Exercises [online]. Available at: www.getselfhelp.co.uk/docs/gilbert-compassion-handout.pdf (accessed March 2024).

Gire J (2014) **H**ow death imitates life: cultural influences on conceptions of death and dying. *Developmental Psychology and Culture 6 (2).*

Gross JJ, Cartensen LL, Pasupathi M, Tsai J, Skorpen CG & Hsu AY (1997) Emotion and ageing*: Experience, express*ion, and control. Psychology and Aging 12 (4) 590-599. doi: 10.1037//0882-7974.12.4.590.

Hamill M & Mahony K (2011) The long goodbye: Cognitive Analytic Therapy with carers of people with dementia. British Journal of Psychotherapy 27 (3) 292-304.

Hepple J & Sutton L (2004) Cognitive Analytic Therapy and Later Life. Hove: Brunner Routledge.

Hepple J & Sutt*on L (2004) Cognitive Analytic Therapy in Later Life. Routledge.*

*Hershfield H, Mikels JA, Sullivan SJ & Carstensen LL (*2008) Poignancy: Mixed emotional experience in the face of meaningful endings. Journal of Personality and Social Psychology 94 (1) 158–167. doi:10.1037/0*022-3514.94.*1.**1**58.

Hershfield HE, Scheibe S, Sims TL, Carstensen LL (2013) When feeling bad can be good: Mixed emotions benefit physical health across adulthood. Social Psychological and Personality Science 4 (1) 54–61. doi:10.1177/1948550612444616.

Hesse H (1952) Hymn to Old Age. Penguin Random House.

Hjelmborg J, Iachine I, Skytthe A, Vaupel JW, McGue M, Koskenvuo M, Kaprio J, Peders*en NL, Christensen K (*2**00**6) Genetic influence on human life*span and longevity. Human Genetics 119 (3) 312–21. doi: 10.1007/s00439-006-0144-y.*

Hofstede G, Minkov M & Hofstede GJ (2010) Cultures and Organizations: Software of t*he Mind: Intercultural* Cooperation and Its Importance for Survival, 3rd edition. *Maidenhead: McGraw-Hill.*

Hollis J (2006) Finding Meaning in the Second H*alf of Life. Penguin, Random House, New York.*

*Houlfort N et al (*2015) The role of passion for work and need sa*tisfaction in psy*chological adjustment to retirement. Vocational Behaviour 88 p84-94.

*Hulme A (2020) N*ext Steps: Life transitions and retirement in the twenty first century. Re*port for Calouste Gulbenkian Foundation.*

*Hummert ML, Garstka TA, Shaner JL & Strahm S (1994) Stereotypes of the elde*rly held by young, middle-aged, and elde*rly adults. J Geron*tol. 49 (5) 240-9. doi: 10.1093/geronj/49.5.p240. PMID: 8056949

Jeffreys B, Almroth-Wright I & Stafford S. 'Ofsted: Head Teacher's Family Blam*es Death on School Inspectio*n Pressure'. BBC, 21 March 2023. Avai*lable at: www.bbc.co.uk/news/uk-england-berkshire-65021154 (accessed March 2024).*

Johnston, D. (2000). A series of cases of dement*ia presenting with PTSD symptoms in World War II veterans. Journal of the* American .Geriatrics Society. *48(1): 70-72.*

Kerr IB & Ryle A (2006) An introduction to the psychotherapies. Cognitive Analytic Therapy (pp. 273). Milt*on Keynes: Open University Press.*

*Kinder, George. (1999) The Sev*en Stages of Money Maturity: Understanding the Spirit *and Value of Money in Your Life. Penguin, Random H*ouse Canada.

Kitwood T (1997) Dement*ia reconsidered: The person comes first. Berkshire, UK Open University* Press.

Kubicek B et al (2011) Psychological well-being in retirement: The effects of personal and gendered contextual resources. Journal of Occupational Health Psychology.

Leiman *M (2002) Toward semiotic dialogism the rol*e of sign mediation in the dialogical sel*f. Theory and P*sychology 12 221-235.

MacKinlay E (2010) Age*ing and Spirituality Across Faiths and Cultures. Philadelphia, PA: Jessica K*ingsley Publishers.

Martinez-Clavera C, James S, Bowditch E & Kuruvilla T (2017) Delayed-onset post-traumatic stress disorder symptoms in dementia. Progress in Neurology and Psychiatry 21 (3) 26-31.

Maslow AH (1943) A theory of human motivation. Psychological Review 50(4) 370-396.

Mather M & Carstensen LL (2005) Aging and motivated cognition: The positivity effect in attention and memory. Trends in Cognitive Sciences 9 (10) 496–502. doi:10.1016/j.tics.2005.08.005.

Mather M (2012) The emotion paradox in the aging brain. Annals of the New York Academy of Sciences 1251 33–49. doi:10.1111/j.1749-6632.2012.06471.x

Mather M (2020) Commentary on aging and positive mood: Longitudinal neurobiological and cognitive correlates. The American Journal of Geriatric Psychiatry 28 (9) 957–958. doi:10.1016/j.jagp.2020.06.005.

Mattinson J (1988) Work, Love and Marriage: The impact of unemployment. Duckworth. London.

McBride K (2008) Will I Ever Be Good Enough? Healing the daughters of narcissistic mothers. Atria.

McCormick, E. (2017) Change for the Better. Personal development through practical psychotherapy (5th ed). London: SAGE Publications.

McCormick E (1990) Change for the Better: Self-Help through practical psychotherapy (1st Edition). Harper Collins: London.

McCormick E (2017) Change for the Better. Personal development through practical psychotherapy (5th ed). London: SAGE Publications.

McCormick E (2017) Change for the Better: Self-help through practical psychotherapy (5th Edition). Sage: London.

McCormick E (2017) Change for the Better: Self-help through practical psychotherapy (5th Edition). Sage: London.

McDougal, J (1989) Theatres of the Body: A Psychoanalytic Approach to Psychosomatic Illness. Free Association Books, London, UK.

McDougal J (1986) Theatres of the Mind: Illusion and truth on the psychoanalytical stage. Free Association Books: London, UK.

Merck (2021) Embracing Carers™, a global initiative led by Merck. Carer Wellbeing Index Study. Available at: https://www.embracingcarers.com/wp-content/uploads/Global-Carer-Well-Being-Index-Report_FINAL.pdf (accessed Apr 2024).

Mittal, D., Torres, R., Abashidze, A., & Jimerson, N. (2001). Worsening of post-traumatic stress disorder symptoms with cognitive decline: case series. Journal of Geriatric Psychiatry and Neurology 14(1): 17-20.

Mroczek DK & Kolarz CM (1998) The effect of age on positive and negative affect: A developmental perspective on happiness. Journal of Personality and Social Psychology 75 (5) 1333-1349. doi: 10.1037/0022-3514.75.5.1333.

OECD (2020) Wide gap in pension benefits between men and women [online]. Available at: www.oecd.org/gender/data/wide-gap-in-pension-benefits-between-men-and-women.htm (accessed March 2024).

Officer A, Thiyagarajan JA, Schneiders ML, Nash P, de la Fuente-Núñez V. Ageism, Healthy Life Expectancy and Population Ageing: How Are They Related? (2020) International Journal of Environmental Research and Public Health 17 (9) 3159. https://doi.org/10.3390/ijerph17093l5

ONS (2022) People aged 65 years and over in employment, UK. January to March 2022, April to June 2022. Labour Force Survey.

ONS. Data and analysis from Census 2021. National life tables – life expectancy in the UK Statistical Bulletins.

Osborne J (2009) Commentary on retirement, identity and Erikson's Developmental Stage Model. Canadian Journal of Aging 28(4) 295-301.

Passarino G, De Rango F, Montesanto A (2016) Human longevity: Genetics or lifestyle? It takes two to tango. Immun Ageing 13 (12) doi: 10.1186/s12979-016-0066-z.

Peltier M. R., Verplaetse T. L., Roberts W., Moore K., Burke C., Marotta P. L., et al. . (2020). Changes in excessive alcohol use among older women across the menopausal transition: a longitudinal analysis of the study of women's health across the nation. Biol. Sex Differ. 11, 37. 10.1186/s13293-020-00314-7 - DOI - PMC - PubMed

Pfeiffer E (1977) Psychopathology and social pathology. In: JE. Birren & KW Schaie (eds.) Handbook of the Psychology of Aging (pp 650-671). Van Nostrand Reinhold.

Potter, S. (2020). Therapy with a Map: A Cognitive Analytic Therapy Approach to Helping Relationships. West Sussex: Pavilion Publishing.

Potter S (2020) Therapy with a map. A Cognitive Analytic Approach to Helping Relationships. *West Sussex: Pavilion Publishing and Media.*

Potter S (2020) Therapy with a Map. Shoreham-by-Sea: Pavilion Publishing and Media.

Potter S (2022) Talking with a Map. Shoreham-by-Sea: Pavilion Publishing and Media.

Qureshi SU, Kimbrell T, Pyne JM, Magruder KM, Hudson TJ, Petersen NJ et al. (2010) Greater prevalence and incidence of dementia in older veterans with posttraumatic stress disorder. The Journal of the American Geriatric Society 58, 1627–1633.

Regier DA, Myers JK, Kramer M, Robins LN, Blazer DG, Hough RL, Eaton WW & Locke BZ (1984) The NIMH Epidemiologic Catchment Area program. Historical context, major objectives, and study population characteristics. Archives of General Psychiatry 41 (10) 934-941. doi:10.1001/archpsyc.1984.01790210016003.

Reitzes D et al (2004) The transition to retirement: strategies and factors that influence retirement adjustment. International Journal of Aging and Human Development 59 (1).

Richardson V & Kilty K (2008) Gender differences in mental health before and after retirement. Journal of Women and Ageing 7 (1-2).

Rilke, Rainer Maria (1905) *Book of Hours: Love Poems to God. Translated Barrows*, A. and Macy, J. p. 165. Northwestern University Press, Evanston, Illinois.

Ruzich M, Looi J, & Robertson M (2005) Delayed Onset of Posttraumatic Stress Disorder Among Male Combat Veterans: A Case Series. The American Journal of Geriatric Psychiatry Volume 13, Issue 5, May 2005, Pages 424-427

Ryle A & Kerr I (2020) Introducing Cognitive Analytic Therapy: Principles and Practice of a relational approach to mental health (2nd ed.). Chichester: Wiley.

Ryle A & Kerr I (2020) Introducing Cognitive Analytic Therapy: Principles and Practice of a relational approach to mental health (2nd ed.). Chichester: Wiley.

Ryle A & Kerr I (2020) Introducing Cognitive Analytic Therapy: Principles and practice of a relational approach to mental health (2nd ed.). Chichester: Wiley.

Ryle A & Kerr I (2020) Introducing Cognitive Analytic Therapy: Principles and practice of a relational approach to mental health (2nd ed.). Chichester: Wiley.

Sample I (2019) 'Doubting Death: How our brains shield us from mortal truth'. 19 October. The Guardian. Available at: www.theguardian.com/science/2019/oct/19/doubting-death-how-our-brains-shield-us-from-mortal-truth (accessed March 2024).

Samuel J (2018) Grief Works: Stories of life, death and surviving. New York: Scribner.

Segalov M (2022) You have to be thick-skinned: what is it like to lose the status of a top job? 25 October. The Guardian.

Shallcross AJ, Ford BQ, Floerke VA & Mauss IB (2012) Getting better with age: the relationship between age, acceptance, and negative affect. Journal of Personality and Social Psychology. Advance online publication. doi: 10.1037/a0031180.

Shallcross AJ, Ford BQ, Floerke VA & Mauss IB (2013) 'Getting better with age: The relationship between age, acceptance, and negative affect': Correction to Shallcross et al (2013). Journal of Personality and Social Psychology 105 (4) 718–719. https://doi.org/10.1037/a0034225

Snowdon D (2008) Aging with Grace: What the nun study teaches us about leading longer, healthier, and more meaningful lives. Random House Publishing Group.

Stevens, Anthony (1994) Jung: A Very Short Introduction. New York. Oxford University Press.

Stroebe M, Schut H & Boerner K (2017) Cautioning health-care professionals: Bereaved persons are misguided through the stages of grief. Journal of Death and *Dying 74 (4).*

*Sze JA, Gyurak A, Good*kind MS & Levenson RW (2012) Greater emotional empathy and prosocial behaviour in late life. Emotion (Washing, DC) 12 (5) 1129-1140. doi: 10.1037/a0025011.

Takata H, Suzuki M, Ishii T, Sekiguchi S, Iri H (1987) Influence of major histocompatibility *complex region genes on human* longevity among Okinawan-Japanese centenarians and nonagenarians. Lancet 1987 Oct 10;2(8563):824-6. doi: 10.1016/s0140-6736(87)91015-4.

Thich Nhat Hanh (2012) Fear: Essential wisdom for getting through *the storm. Rider: UK.*

Tokarczuk O (2019) The Tender Narrator [online]. Available at: www.nobelprize.org/prizes/literature/2018/tokarczuk/lecture/ (accessed March 2024).

Ubel PA, Loewenstein G, Hershey J, et al (2001) Do nonpatients underestimate the quality of life associated *with chronic health conditions because of a fo*cusing illusion? Med Decis Making 21 (3) 190–9.

Ubel PA, Loewenstei*n G, Schwarz N, Smith D (2005) Misimagining the unimaginable: the disability paradox and health care decisio*n making. Health Psychol 24 (4) (Suppl.) S57–62, July.

United For All Ages (2017) A country for all ages: ending age apartheid in Brexit Britain [o*nline]. Available at:* www.eldersvoice.org.uk/wp-content/uploads/2022/11/Ending-Age-Apartheid-Report.pdf (accessed March 2024).

Vaillant, G. E. (2002). Aging well: Surprising guideposts to a happier life from the Landmark Harvard Study of Adult Developm*ent. B*oston: Little, Brown and Company.

van Achterberg M, Rohrbaugh R, & Southwick S (2001) Emergence of PTSD in trauma survivors with dementia. Journal of Clinical Psychiatry, Mar; 62 (3):206-7

Van Der Kolk B (2015) The Body Keeps the Score: *Brain, mind, and* body in the healing of trauma. Penguin: UK.

Wagstyl S (2022) 'Most Britons have "no idea" about their retirement income'. Financial Times.

Wang M & S*hi J (2014) Ps*ychological research on retirement. Annual Review of Psych*ology 65 209-233.*

WHO (2021) Ageism is a Global Challenge: UN [online]. Available at: www.who.int/news/item/18-03-2021-ageism-is-a-global-challenge-un (accessed March 2024).

WHO (2022) Ageing and Health [online]. Available at: www.who.int/news-room/fact-sheets/detail/ageing-and-health (accessed March 2024).

Winnicott D (1960) Ego distortion in terms if True and False self. In: The Maturational Processes and the Facilitating Environment. Routledge, UK.

World Health Organisation (2020) Dementia [online]. Available at*: www.who.int/*news-room/fact-sheets/detail/dementia (accessed March 2024).

*Yaffe K, Vittinghoff E, Lindquis*t K, Barnes D, Covinsky KE, Neylan T et al. (2010) Posttraumatic stress disorder and risk of dementia among US veterans. Arc*hives of General P*sychiatry 67, 608–613.

Zelenski E (2022) How to Retire Happy, Wild and Free. VIP Books, Edmonton, Canada